MAKING THE CUT

Making the Cut

How Cosmetic Surgery is
Transforming our Lives

Anthony Elliott

REAKTION BOOKS

For Charles Lemert

Published by Reaktion Books Ltd
33 Great Sutton Street
London EC1V ODX, UK
www.reaktionbooks.co.uk

First published 2008

Printed and bound in Great Britain
by Cromwell Press, Trowbridge, Wiltshire

British Library Cataloguing in Publication Data
Elliott, Anthony
  Making the cut : how cosmetic surgery is transforming our lives
  1. Surgery, Plastic - Social aspects
  I. Title
  306.4'613

ISBN-13: 978 1 86189 371 0

Contents

Introduction

In the new economy nothing is more sexy than surgery. From Botox and lipo to tummy tucks and mini-facelifts, the number of cosmetic surgery operations undertaken around the globe has soared recently, as consumers spend more and more on themselves in the search for sex appeal and artificial beauty. In a society in which celebrity is divine, information technology rules, new ways of working predominate and people increasingly judge each other on first impressions, cosmetic enhancements of the body have become all the rage.

Increasingly, cosmetic surgical culture goes all the way down in our society. One recent European survey found that most women now expect to have cosmetic surgery at some point in their lifetime.[1] Another survey, this time American, discerned that more than half of businessmen would undergo the surgeon's knife in order to advance their professional careers. Makeover culture for the rest of us, it seems, is now just part and parcel of daily life. Cosmetic surgery is simply another lifestyle choice, alongside fashion, fitness and therapy.

In *Making the Cut*, I want to examine how society goes about the making and remaking of cosmetic surgical culture. In chapter One I begin by analysing the dynamics of cosmetic surgical culture in relation to society, culture, economics and politics. A life lived in the shadow of the

7

pursuit of lipo, I argue, is one deeply conditioned by three crucial forces – and each is as cultural as it is structural. The first concerns celebrity: the impact of changing notions of fame is more and more central to people's decisions to undertake cosmetic procedures and surgical alterations of the body. From the endless media scrutinizing of celebrity bodies – such as Paris Hilton, Angelina Jolie and Nicole Kidman – to the mesmerizing cultural influence of reality TV programmes such as *Extreme Makeover* and *The Swan*, increasing numbers are following the cult of celebrity straight to the operating theatre. This development is the outcome of a complex set of transformations from fame to celebrity, and its conditions and consequences are examined in chapter Two.

The second factor driving cosmetic surgical culture is consumerism. Buying beauty – changing one's looks, personal makeover, body enhancements – is now a central part of life in the expensive cites of the West, primarily undertaken by women but also increasingly by men. From age-reversing skin creams and cosmetic dentistry to Botox and breast augmentation, the marketing and packaging of artificially enhanced beauty are now fundamental to the selling of 'the successful life'. In this respect, an acquisitive individualism concerned with the buying of more and more goods – has been intensified. Today savvy consumers are not only focused on the purchase of select goods or services, but they also compulsively purchase the improvement of the self through the buying of enhanced body parts. In this sense, today's consuming identities of cosmetic surgical culture have taken on an addictive cast. The combined weight of the consumer industry and rampant consumerism has shaped cosmetic surgical culture to its roots. Chapter Three explores some of the ways in which the development of consumerism and the consumer industries has affected people's conceptions of their bodies and identities as experienced in cosmetic surgical culture.

The third factor driving cosmetic surgical culture follows from the others, but is rarely explicitly considered in discussions of the topic. It concerns the new economy heralded by globalization; that is, how the rapid pace of economic change today shapes wider cultural imperatives concerning employment adaptability as well as flexibility of identity. My argument is that the new economy spawned by globalization intrudes traumatically in the emotional lives of people – with many scrambling to adjust to today's routine corporate redundancies. Chapter Four focuses on the dramatic changes now occurring in the global electronic economy and on the ways in which corporate lay-offs, downsizings and offshorings are affecting people's sense of identity, life and work. For the price of jobs potentially downsized or lost as a result of the new economy, as Louis Uchitelle and N. R. Kleinfield comment, is 'the most acute job insecurity since the Depression. And this in turn has produced an unrelenting angst that is shattering people's notions of work and self and the very promise of tomorrow.'[2] Many have reacted to this sense of social dislocation and economic insecurity – what I term today's pervasive sense of *ambient fear* – by turning to forms of extreme reinvention in general and cosmetic surgical culture in particular. Many are calculating that a freshly purchased face-lift or suctioning of fat through liposuction is the best route to improved lives, careers and relationships.

For the most part, it has been the media that have drawn attention to these transformations in a general way. Newspaper headlines report the rising tide of job insecurity in the new economy, and of practices of extreme reinvention that individuals are undertaking as a consequence. The *Wall Street Journal* runs the headline 'Plastic Surgery Wooing Patients Hoping To Move Up Career Ladder'.[3] The *New York Times* leads with 'Sometimes, Nips and Tucks Can Be Career Moves'.[4] The *Boston Globe* reports 'A

New Wrinkle in the Rat Race'.[5] The magazine *Canadian Business* notes 'Knife Guys Finish First'.[6] *Personnel Today* highlights 'Plastic Surgery Could Be the Key To Rejuvenating a Sagging Career'.[7] And an Australian newspaper recently ran the headline '$20,000 Face Buys a New Job', with the sub-heading 'It's Better than Renovating the Kitchen'.[8] All these media reports note the broader connections between business and beauty, commerce and the cosmetic. All place an emphasis on artificial beauty and the surgical enhancement of the body as a means of adapting to the pressures of corporate life and the global economy. In each case the analysis is broad, the detail sketchy. By contrast, the aim of this book is to analyse cosmetic surgical culture and its relation to the new economy of advanced globalization rigorously and in detail.

Reference to the 'new economy' has become a stereotype within recent discussions of globalization, and I should at the outset clarify its meaning as used throughout this book. The new economy, as I deploy the term, refers to the emergence of computer-based production technology, especially in the service, finance and communication sectors; the spread of new information technologies that underpin spatially dispersed global production and consumption; and new ways of organizing work, primarily around the imperatives of adaptability and flexibility.[9] All these features of the new economy have spelt rapid change throughout both public and private life, and probably nowhere more so than in people's fears over self-worth, the splintering of personal identity and the fragmentation of family life. Indeed, it is in the shift from the traditional work contract (long-term job security, orderly promotions, longevity-linked pay and pensions) to the new work deal (short-term contracts, job hopping and options shopping, high risk-taking) that a new kind of fear nests. Fear of future uncertainties – work, relationships, life itself – is what drives many in contemporary societies, I argue, to make sense of such social dislocation through cosmetic surgical culture. Of course, such reactions to current global transformations are still relatively small in scale; and I do not contend that the new economy represents the whole economy. But the new economy, as Richard Sennett rightly argues, 'does exert a profound moral and normative force as a cutting-edge standard for how the larger economy should evolve'.[10] For this reason alone, there ought to be value in setting out the idea of cosmetic surgery culture in a rather more novel context, one that might loosely be portrayed as both creation and reaction to the global electronic economy.

I should at this point tell the reader something about the kind of research I have undertaken in writing this book. Throughout *Making the Cut*, I have drawn extensively from newspaper, magazine and online contributions, as well as debates over the topic of cosmetic surgery, to develop my argument. A sceptical reader of the book might well question the method, or wonder why I pay so much attention to the experiences of ordinary people as portrayed by the media. The answer is straightforward. Some of the most telling examples of cosmetic surgical culture and its deep affinities with the global economy are to be found in the media, and in this respect it is true to say that journalistic accounts of cosmetic surgery are for the most part more probing than many academic studies published to date. In using the media as a research resource, I have tried to read widely, citing articles from the *New York Times* and *Time* on the one hand and local dailies like the *Adelaide Advertiser* or management magazines on the other. The result, I hope, reflects the reach of cosmetic surgical culture, as well as the intensity of both its local and global dynamism.

But it is the people I've interviewed over recent years – the numerous surgeons and cosmetic surgery patients – that inform my argument and tell the narratives of *Making the Cut*. In this regard, the book grants particular privilege to the investigation of the personal or subjective as a means of better grasping a complicated social phenomenon. It is especially the emotional contradictions, psychic tensions and interpersonal difficulties in people's experience of their identities and bodies as refracted through cosmetic surgical culture that informs my argument about the wider import of the new economy and globalization. To that extent, as with my previous book *The New Individualism: The Emotional Costs of Globalization* written with Charles Lemert, I have taken the liberty of speaking for the people I have interviewed through the writing of fictionalized stories. This I have done partly as a means of protecting or disguising individual identities. But, equally significantly, the fictional stories I tell serve as a means of condensing the specifics of narrative told to me during my many hours of listening to people. Thus, in compressing several voices into one, I have tried to capture more precisely what is going on in people's minds, and to grasp something of the concrete experience of cosmetic surgical culture.

Finally, the reader will find social theories applied to, or juxtaposed with, the discussions of an individual's understanding of cosmetic surgical culture. As a professional sociologist, I have no hesitation in doing so. For one thing, it is my view that the sociological imagination – both professional and practical – is enriched through the mingling of interview data, journalistic accounts, media interviews, sociological perspectives and social theories. Yet in adopting this approach to the writing of the book, my central aim is to establish a connection between critics of cosmetic surgical culture on the one hand and scholars of globalization and the new economy on the other. For the most part, these groups have had little, if anything, to say to each other. But to the extent that my argument in *Making the Cut* is correct, the interconnections between commerce and the cosmetic are increasingly fundamental to the new economy. My argument is that this problematic set of relationships – between cosmetic surgical culture and the global makeover industries – requires rigorous analysis.

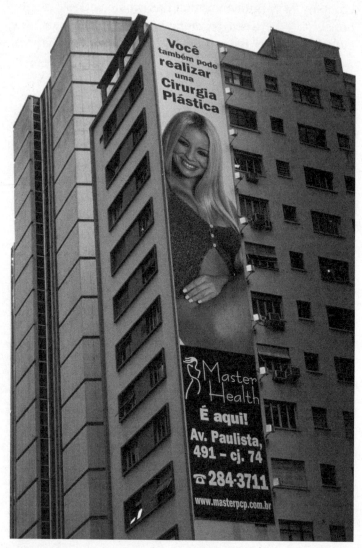

A 2002 advertisement for cosmetic surgery in Brazil, showing
Juliana Dornelles Borges, who became 'Miss Brazil' after nineteen
cosmetic surgery operations.

Chapter 1

Drastic Plastic: The Rise of Cosmetic Surgical Culture

Leaving my home in Bristol to catch the early commuter train to London, today is my first day of interviewing cosmetic and plastic surgeons working on Harley Street. After months of analysing both popular and academic writing on cosmetic surgery, I am expecting to enter a world blending economic privilege with advanced techno-logy, a world of instant self-reinvention realized through skin-tightening procedures like Thermage and surgical interventions like liposuction or autologous fat transfer. I am expecting a highly polished welcome; a slick, stylized clinic; a narcissistic obsession with the stretching, pumping and tucking of skin for the purpose of beautification. But when I arrive at Dr David Hargraves's office, none of this seems apparent. The waiting room is colourless, almost drab. There are no pictures of people – celebrities, models – who have surgically transformed themselves on display. And Dr Hargraves's secretary doesn't seem to be expect-ing me. This, I tell myself, doesn't look promising.

Dr Hargraves works in the field of plastic, reconstruc-tive and rehabilitation surgery. After his secretary locates my appointment and someone from reception escorts me through to his office, my initial thought is that I've chosen the wrong surgeon to interview. Looking around this most sober and serene office, I imagine that Dr Hargraves works principally in the public sector, dealing with injured patients that require reconstructive and other specialist procedures. As vitally important as such work is, this isn't my research brief. I'm concerned with the dramatic rise in the number of Westerners increasingly concerned with and insecure about appearance. I especially want to know what drives people to a personal makeover through cosmetic surgical culture.

Enter David Hargraves, wearing an open-neck shirt with navy jacket, carrying a bundle of papers, looking engrossed in his own reverie. A quietly spoken man, he shakes my hand somewhat nervously, gesturing for me to sit down and begin the interview. Two thoughts flash through my mind. The first is that he probably hasn't been interviewed before, and my general impression is that getting him to talk might be really difficult. The second is that he looks of advancing years, maybe late fifties, and clearly isn't using his own face as advertising space for the wonders of cosmetic surgery.

I try to put these thoughts to one side, and ask him to describe his professional history. He tells me that, for many years, he worked largely for the National Health Service, as a reconstructive surgeon. Much of his work centred on burns and related injury patients. During the late 1980s he started to see more private patients requesting cosmetic surgery. This was a trend that escalated throughout the 1990s, and today the bulk of his work encompasses aesthetic, or cosmetic, surgery. I ask him why he's moved to working with generally healthy patients whose prime motivation is to improve their looks. His answer is disarmingly direct. Such work, he tells me, is financially highly lucrative. I decide things are looking up for my research.

Most of his patients, Hargraves tells me, are women. But he has been seeing an increasing number of men for cosmetic surgery too. 'What drives people to cosmetic surgery?', I ask. 'Many factors', comments Hargraves.

It's about improving life, and especially business opportunities. Many of my patients work in highly demanding business environments, in which flexibility and adaptability really count, and in which appearance is all important. These are professional people, responding to very pressured demands, who are being judged by their clientele in the first few seconds of meeting. One of the greatest worries people have today is of looking tired – of being judged by an employer not up for the job.

Such worries may not, of course, figure as the most urgent problems confronting modern society. There are more pressing matters to worry about than the onset of crow's feet, patchy skin or stomach bulges. But worry people do, and increasingly so. According to Hargraves, the very conditions that have brought the possibility of longer life into being (advances in medicine and new technologies) have also made possible the rise of makeover culture.

Cosmetic surgery and societal demands for it are directly connected to the welfare of the economy. When times are good and there's increased economic prosperity, we witness a rise in demand for face-lifts.

For Hargraves, the economy rules.

Consider, then, this economistic idea of cosmetic surgical culture, one based on the prosperity of the economy, with the following story of a professional women – I will call her Amanda Brown – as relayed to me by Hargraves. Amanda Brown had undergone a breast enlargement procedure with Hargraves a few years before. Brown, a tall, attractive women in her early thirties, said that she wanted implants at the time of initial consultation because she had long been unhappy with the size and shape of her breasts. She requested a cup size of full c, and Hargraves agreed to undertake the procedure. Brown, he tells me, was generally pleased with her breast implants – though, as with many women, it took her some considerable time to adjust to the hard, swollen feeling of her redesigned body.

Recently, as it happens, Brown returned to Dr Hargraves's consulting rooms. She returned, he tells me, to request jumbo implants – DD cup size. Her reason for requesting a second breast augmentation, or rather the justification she gave at the time, was that she felt she hadn't fully reached her personal potential. Hargraves comments that he was initially suspicious, and probed further her motivations. The true reason: her husband. Hargraves tells me that Brown's husband is the CEO of a leading financial institution in London, and that it was very important to him that his wife 'turned the heads of others' when the couple were socializing and entertaining. Good for his image, good for business. According to Brown's frank admission, her husband had been always attracted by her slender body and small waist – but, increasingly, he wanted her redesigned with large breasts. In short, he wanted Barbie.

Amanda Brown, driven by the emotional and sexual demands of her husband, is far from alone in contemplating the Barbie look. More and more, the surgically enhanced body of what Alex Kuczynski calls 'tits on sticks' is all the rage. As Kuczynski writes:

> The ideal breast itself is a model straight out of adolescence: a firm, smooth globe, the perfect marriage of cone and sphere, topped with a tiny rosebud of a nipple, one that has not been marred and dimpled by the application of infants' suckling lips. It is, of course, rather unusual for a woman who is slender on the bottom half to have enough body fat to sustain large breasts on the top. Yet so many American women choose to emulate this ideal – and so many men appear to admire it – that it points to our ever-growing love for the artificial over the organic.[1]

It may, of course, be illegible to Brown that a love for the artificial over the organic is at the root of her search for 'perfect breasts'. It is clearly not illegible to Dr Hargraves, who entertained serious reservations about performing this second breast augmentation. But such reservations, he points out, are difficult to sustain. If he didn't perform the procedure, he reasons, another London surgeon would. But whatever these ethical ambiguities, I am most struck by the story's link to the sense of instant self-reinvention today. If it is a love for the artificial over the organic that influences Brown's decision to redesign her body, this is a love that goes all the way down to the very fabric of our cultural and economic complexity as a society. If artificially enhanced beauty and business are near neighbours, and Dr Hargraves certainly believes that Brown wanted the implants to placate her husband and his business ambitions, this is because instant self-reinvention fits in perfectly with the flexibility, flow and flux that mark society today.

From London to New York, Madrid to Melbourne, Tehran to Singapore, trade in cosmetic surgery is soaring. Botox, collagen fillers, breast implants, microdermabrasion, mini-face-lifts: extreme reinvention is all the rage. Today, phrases such as 'liquid lifestyles' and 'flexible futures' describe not only the very structure of a global economy that has brought profound change in contemporary organizational structures, but also a set of emergent obsessions and fears that people increasingly experience in trying to alter their identities, personalities and bodies.

Cosmetic surgical culture is one of excess, fear, disposability anxieties and melancholia. Consider, for example, the following media reports, all of which highlight the myriad ways in which the combined forces of globalization, high technology and the new economy are shaping people's demands for instant self-reinvention through cosmetic surgery.

According to US government statistics, growing numbers of people are seeking cosmetic surgery to get ahead in the workplace. Cosmetic procedures for men have more than doubled in the US over recent years, and surgeons have noted a dramatic rise in the number of requests from business executives, lawyers, estate agents and airline pilots, among others.[2]

'A growing number of professionals', reports the *Boston Globe*, 'are visiting image consultants and even plastic surgeons in a quest to get an edge on younger competitors for jobs and promotions in a still-tough economy.' Executive Marilyn V. Santiesteban, who is reported as having undergone a personal makeover, comments: 'I believe that a professional image should be updated as frequently as a resumé'. Business executives wanting new, younger looks are signing up for standard procedures of nose jobs, liposuction, breast augmentation, eyelid lifts and face lifts. Dr Joel Feldman, from the Massachusetts General Hospital, comments that people's increased demand for plastic surgery is 'because they believe they'll be received better at work and feel better about themselves at the same time'.[3]

In early 2007 Lebanon's First National Bank rolled out a new product, which is unique in the Middle East: a loan for plastic surgery. The product's launch was delayed because of Israel's war against the Hizbollah movement in Lebanon, but when the loan and advertising campaign began there were billboards of a young blond model posted across the country. George Nasr, head of the bank's marketing department, estimates that the number of cosmetic procedures has doubled in Lebanon since 2000, and recent figures estimate that the industry is worth between $25 and $30 million.[4]

A recent study by the Connecticut-based wealth research firm Prince & Associates says that 81 per cent of Americans with a net worth of more than $10 million are planning to go under the knife for cosmetic plastic surgery over the next two years.[5]

These media reports on cosmetic surgery trends are, in various respects, sociologically suggestive about the broader contours of modern culture. It is useful to contextualize such media coverage, however, by widening the discussion to encompass the rise of cosmetic surgical culture in contemporary societies.

By any standards, cosmetic surgical culture is a massive global business. In the United States alone, it is estimated that cosmetic surgery is an industry generating $15 to $20 billion a year.[6] Whilst this may fall short of other beauty businesses, such as the $25 billion-a-year cosmetics industry and the more than $30 billion-a-year diet industry, cosmetic plastic surgery is the fastest growing beauty business in the world today. For example, in early 2007 the American Society of Plastic Surgeons announced that some 11 million cosmetic plastic surgery procedures had been performed in the US during the previous twelve months, a figure up some 7 per cent from 2005. This contrasts sharply to the 2 million cosmetic surgical procedures undergone by Americans in 1988, a contrast highlighting that cosmetic surgical culture appeals not simply to the fashion-conscious but to Americans in general.

At the same time, the appetite for surgical enhancement has grown rapidly, such that redesigned body parts are now among the most erotically alluring commodities in these early years of the twenty-first century. Culture has no doubt always been concerned with sex, its representations and signs; but today we have a whole society held in thrall to the drastic plastic of labial rejuvenation (in which the vagina is snipped and re-sculpted), breast nipple enhancement and buttock implants. Our cultural obsession shows in the numbers. According to the American Society of Plastic Surgeons, surgical procedures increased in the years 2005–6 as follows: breast augmentation by 13 per cent, lower body lifts by 19 per cent, vaginal rejuvenation by 30 per cent and pectoral implants by 50 per cent. In addition, in 2006 surgeons of the Society also performed more than 9 million non-invasive procedures, an increase of 8 per cent on 2005. The top five minimally invasive procedures were Botox (4.1 million), chemical peel (1.1 million), laser hair removal (887,000), microdermabrasion (817,000) and hyaluronic acid fillers (778,000).

Perhaps not surprisingly, women easily outspend men on cosmetic surgery. I say 'perhaps' in this context because the past few decades have witnessed significant moves towards gender equality throughout contemporary Western societies, as well as the spread of more progressive values governing sexual politics in general. Yet in the contemporary world many people would not contest the ongoing reality and social force of gender hierarchy; indeed, many feminists view the upheavals of globalization as fundamental to women's sense of disempowerment as lived in terms of unequal gender relations. One recent account of such ongoing distortions to our sexual politics focuses on the rise of 'raunch culture', the contemporary trend for soft-porn styling in everything from thongs to lap-dancing classes, Playboy T-shirts to silicone implants.[7] In any case, and whatever the cause of the massive discrepancy between the sexes in terms of cosmetic consumerism, women account for roughly 90 per cent of cosmetic surgical patients in the United States. Moreover, American women are today spending approximately 55 per cent more on cosmetic surgical procedures than they did in 2000. That said, it is certainly evident too that men are more and more drawn into the dominant structures of cosmetic surgical culture. There are, of course, no end of media reports of men engaging in surgical enhancements of the body to improve their careers in, say, modelling, sports and the media. But a more measured account of the rising numbers of men undergoing the surgeon's knife comes from the figures for 2006 released by the American Society of Plastic Surgeons pertaining to a surge in the following procedures: since 2000 thigh lifts saw an increase of 180 per cent and tummy tucks of 165 per cent. The biggest increases in men's use of cosmetic surgical culture can be found in various non-invasive procedures, which require less healing time than surgical procedures and, thus, less time away from the work environment. Botox remains the most popular minimally invasive procedure in the US for men, and its use has gone up by more than 200 per cent since 2000. Likewise, microdermabrasion is also favoured by American men, and its use has witnessed a rise of 112 per cent since 2000.

Cosmetic surgical culture across the United States, however, is far more complex and differentiated than these figures from the American Society of Plastic Surgeons would suggest. For one thing, the American Society of Plastic Surgeons – while it is the largest organization of board-certified plastic surgeons in the world – comprises approximately 6,000 members. However, many patients seeing cosmetic and plastic surgeons in the US consult experts from other organizations. There are not authoritative statistics on this, although some of the relevant organizations in this context would include the American Society for Aesthetic Plastic Surgery, Cosmetic Surgery USA and the American Academy of Cosmetic Surgery. Such organizations subscribe to quite different professional cosmetic and surgical guidelines and procedures for patients, and physicians are likely to recommend or use different products according to their professional membership.

Similar nip and tuck trends are evident throughout the United Kingdom. As with data from the US, statistics pertaining to the rise of cosmetic surgical culture in the UK are far from authoritative or conclusive. Yet to get a fix on the growing numbers of new patients, figures released by the British Association of Aesthetic Plastic Surgeons (BAAPS) are

23

suggestive of broader social trends throughout the expensive, polished cities of the West. BAAPS reported that its surgeons witnessed a 50 per cent increase in 2005 and a 35 per cent increase in 2006 in the number of cosmetic surgery operations undertaken in Britain. At the time of media release, these figures caused quite a public stir in tradition-loving Britain. Probing these reports, however, it transpires that these increased numbers level out at around 40,000 procedures. Some commentators were quick to point out that such numbers are not high if set against the UK population of some 60 million people. Other commentators, however, argued that the figures were indicative of the cosmetic surgery boom if read carefully. This was so because it needs to be borne in mind that BAAPS represents only 200 of the estimated 700 plastic surgeons working in the UK – and thus these figures might be only the tip of the cosmetic surgery iceberg. Moreover, it was pointed out that the BAAPS figures did not include the 'lighter' end of the market – namely, the non-invasive procedures of Botox, collagen fillers and so on.

Even so, a mania for cosmetic surgical culture is certainly reflected in more recent UK studies. For example, market research in 2006 estimated that the UK cosmetic surgery industry is worth more than £528 million annually, an increase of almost 50 per cent on 2005.[8] In this market, the report contends, socio-economic factors are the major drivers for cosmetic surgery in the UK. Nowadays, it is not just vanity or narcissism that propels people to contemplate cosmetic surgery; rather, it is increasingly considered an investment in the future. Low unemployment, increasing disposable incomes and easier access to borrowing throughout the late 1990s and early 2000s in the UK have meant that prospective patients have been able to undertake such 'investments' with ease. A related factor identified by these UK market researchers concerns the astonishing speed of technological change, particularly as regards non-invasive procedures.

Increased sophistication in laser technology is a strong trend and combined treatments involving the use of a number of different types of non-surgical treatment – injectables and peels, as well as the use of cosmeceuticals – is an increasing feature of the market. In terms of surgical procedures, demand in facial surgery, in particular, is being boosted by advancements in minimally invasive techniques, which are encouraging more women to opt for the so-called 'lunch-time lifts'. Recovery times are shorter and consumers can often be back at work shortly after fairly major procedures.[9]

This refers, in the broadest of terms, to the current of cultural experiment we know as instant self-reinvention, and we will be considering the various social implications of this current throughout this book.

As in the UK, the appetite for all things surgical is apparent across Europe. In March 2006 *Time* magazine ran a feature, 'Europe's Extraordinary Makeover', which documented unprecedented numbers of individuals demanding elective cosmetic surgery. Countries such as France, Germany, Spain and Turkey all outstripped Britain in their consumption of the culture of nip and tuck. Interestingly, it is among the younger generation that we find the most passionate embracement of surgical culture.

The main region to see a flourishing of cosmetic surgical culture has been Asia. This has occurred almost overnight. For many decades, Asia lagged behind the West in catching the reinvention craze offered by cosmetic plastic surgery. Today, however, bright young Asians are transfixed by the possibility of remaining young, and of improving their looks, through the surgical fix. From Seoul to Singapore, Asians are experimenting with plastic surgery as never before. In Japan, non-invasive procedures such as Botox and collagen injections have been estimated to be worth US$100 million annually to the top clinics. In Taiwan, more than a million procedures are performed yearly, a figure that has doubled in fewer than five years. In South Korea, surgeons estimate that more than one in ten adults have undergone some form of surgical enhancement to their bodies. And in Thailand cosmetic surgical tours are fashionable.

Asia's recent obsession with cosmetic surgical culture has been inaugurated by the tidal waves of globalization, the new economy and advances in information technology and the media. The emphasis on foregrounding self-rein-vention through surgical enhancement of the body, most obvious in satellite TV and Hollywood culture, is dissemi-nated through a 24/7 mass media, which carries *Cosmetic Surgery Live* and *The Swan* to countries such as Singapore, Thailand and India. There can be little doubt that such globalization of media has proved of central significance in the reshaping of Asia's beauty ideal in recent times. Seduced, captivated and sometimes addicted to Western images of cosmetic surgical culture, more and more Asians desire to remake themselves in the Caucasian mould. But it is not true that this global surgical revolution has trans-formed Asian cultures in a uniform fashion. Whilst the dissemination of cosmetic surgical images across Asia has penetrated deeply into people's understanding of their identities, the adoption of these images – and especially at the level of a translation for demands for surgical enhancement – has been culturally specific. As a report in *Time* reflected on Asia's nip and tuck trend:

> Asians are increasingly asking their surgeons for wider eyes, longer noses and fuller breasts – features not typical of the race. To accommodate such demands, surgeons in the region have had to invent unique tech-niques. The No. 1 procedure by far in Asia is a form of blepharoplasty, in which a crease is created above the eye by scalpel or by needle and thread; in the US, blepharoplasty also ranks near the top, but involves

removing bags and fat around the eyes. Likewise, Westerners use Botox or botulinum toxin, to diminish wrinkles – while in Korea, Japan and Taiwan, Botox is injected into wide cheeks so the muscle will atrophy and the cheeks will shrink.[10]

The essential point here is that although Asia is increasingly drawn into the global economy and its ideological offshoots such as cosmetic surgical culture, such media influences are reworked through new medical technologies to fit with the culturally specific forms of life in Asian society.

Just as cosmetic surgical culture has taken hold in South Korea, Singapore, Thailand and Malaysia, so it has penetrated the fabric of Chinese society. Indeed, recent statistics indicate that China is fast outstripping South Korea as the plastic surgery centre in Asia.[11] Against the backdrop of China's Communist austerity, this is in one sense very surprising, given that cosmetic surgery was banned by Chinese officialdom for some twenty years. Yet today, by contrast, cosmetic surgical culture is one of the fastest growing industries of the Chinese economy. According to recent government figures, the Chinese are spending in excess of US$2.4 billion a year on cosmetic surgery, with more than one million operations performed annually.

That there is a developing link between career success and more liberal attitudes to cosmetic surgery in China is suggested in an *Asia Times* story in 2005 documenting the numbers of well-off Chinese undergoing the plastic surgeon's knife. Here the new face of Chinese cosmetic surgery is presented as individuals 'investing' in themselves – their careers, lifestyles and future life prospects. As this point is developed:

Certainly there are social and economic factors which suggest that the cosmetic industry is a good bet. Wherever you are in the world, the good-looking, thin and tall can expect to earn more than their dowdy, plump or short colleagues – and this in developed countries, often in spite of strict anti-discrimination laws. In China, where employers can freely specify desired appearance in job interviews, the relationship between looks and earnings is, in certain fields at least, even more obvious. The key expression *pinmao duanzhuang*, translating as 'appropriate appearance', appears again and again as a key requirement for jobs involving contact with customers.[12]

The impacts of economic liberalization, Western individualist values and the beginnings of a large-scale shift away from the traditional sexual rigidities of China's Communist era also bear on these emerging attitudes to cosmetic surgery. 'A rapidly expanding and competitive media', the *Asia Times* article notes of China today, 'provides an increasingly receptive audience with the basic message that youth and good looks are central to fulfilment and self-esteem.' But it is career aspirations that remain fundamental to China's nip and tuck trend. As one Chinese client of cosmetic surgery summarized the situation as reported on CBS News:

> It's not just about vanity. In this society, people are judged for jobs and promotions often by how they look. There are reports about people not getting hired because they were deemed too short or too ugly.[13]

Other countries demonstrate similar trends. For example, whilst there are no comprehensive statistics at the present time, the number of cosmetic surgery operations performed in Australia in recent years has soared dramatically. This is certainly true of capital cities such as Sydney and Melbourne, but a rise in the number of Australians demanding remodelling, smoothing and tightening is evident in other cities as well. For example, Adelaide Plastic Surgery

Associates in 2006 reported a 50 per cent jump in the number of its overseas clients. Cosmetic surgery, it would seem, is fast becoming an emerging export for the state of South Australia. And the reasons are not too hard to discern. For a face-lift that would cost AUS$70,000 in London and $25,000 in Sydney costs only $10,000 in Adelaide.

This spread of 'cut-price' cosmetic surgery is not, however, the most interesting aspect of the story. For what's new in the surge of Botox converts and liposuction addicts is the social composition of those undergoing the surgeon's knife. More and more, affluent middle-class professionals are turning to plastic surgery in an effort to retain, or sometimes acquire, youthful looks. The British Association of Aesthetic Plastic Surgeons, for example, reports that professionals have replaced celebrities as the dominant group choosing to reinvent themselves through cosmetic surgery, a trend confirmed by several recent academic studies. Professionals from Jakarta to Singapore to London are going to Australia for cosmetic surgery, managing along the way to combine their cut-price deals with business-class flights and a holiday.

The academic study of cosmetic surgery has not been notable for its insights or controversial arguments. For many years, it was essentially synonymous with the analysis and critique of either nose jobs (rhinoplasty) or facelifts (rhytidectomy).[14] By the 1990s and early 2000s, however, cosmetic surgery was also coming to mean liposuction, breast augumentation, tummy tucks (abdominoplasty), thigh and buttock lifts, eyelid tightening (blephardoplasty), penile enlargements and implants. Cosmetic surgical culture – in magazines, books, radio phone-ins and television – was spreading throughout social life. Yet there were anxieties in the academy as to which procedures should be included in the field, and by definition excluded from it. A conflict broke out over whether collagen and fat injections or Botox properly constituted cosmetic surgery. A more significant quarrel arose over the meanings and differences between cosmetic surgery, referring to the procedures performed on patients who were in general healthy, and plastic surgery, which might include facial reconstruction following a car accident or the reconstruction of a breast after a mastectomy. This was an important area of academic enquiry, although one whose differences the broader public intuitively grasped well enough. Meanwhile, there were protracted and dull debates over whether, say, transgender surgery fell under the umbrella of cosmetic surgical culture or not.

When the academy did finally get around to tackling the more substantive sociological questions arising from cosmetic surgery, it did so, surprisingly, in a very abstract kind of way – primarily through recourse to European social and feminist theories. This was surprising because European social theory, at least in the traditions of thought of post-structuralism and post-feminism, was largely at odds with the images of plastic perfection found in cosmetic surgical culture. The accounts of social and gendered power in post-structural and post-feminist theory, with their high abstractions on language and intertextuality, hardly fits well with the ultra-visual culture of cosmetic surgery – in which women and men are tucked, pumped, stretched, snipped and sculptured. Yet the kind of social theory that began to emerge in the 1990s, in the work of feminists and post-structuralists like Kathy Davis, Virginia L. Blum and Anne Balsamo, was that of cosmetic surgery addicts caught up in and subject to negotiated discourses, mutilated bodies, policed identities and intertextual pathologies.

Notwithstanding such unpromising conceptual starting points, critics have sought to detail an all-inclusive general formula accounting for the rise of cosmetic surgical culture. In *The Beauty Myth*, Naomi Wolf proclaims that the 'current Surgical Age is, like the Victorian medical system, impelled by easy profits'. She argues that capitalism, in its hyper-consumerist phase inaugurated by multinational giants, secretly goes to work on women behind their backs, constructing them as candidates for the lethal and bloody practices of cosmetic surgery. Women are thus condemned to the doomed pursuit of 'beauty', as defined by a system of crazed excess in which surgical interventions are deemed necessary for individuals where no problem actually exists. As Wolf concludes from an Olympian feminist height:

> Whatever the future threatens, we can be fairly sure of this: women in our 'raw' or natural state will continue to be shifted from the category 'woman' to the category 'ugly' and shamed into an assembly-line physical identity.[15]

Like Susan Bordo in her influential *Unbearable Weight*, Kathy Davis's *Reshaping The Female Body: The Dilemma of Cosmetic Surgery* holds that women draw on a repertoire of intersecting cultural discourses pertaining to the body and appearance in order to give narrative substance to their decisions to undergo the surgeon's knife. Drawing on feminist and sociological notions of power, Davis attempts to 'find ways to explore cosmetic surgery as a complex and dilemmatic situation for women: problem and solution, oppression and liberation, all in one'.[16] For Davis, cosmetic surgery inaugurates a new order of discourse in which the notions of choice, decision-making and agency become fundamental to the making and remaking of the female body. This shows up not only in the pain and suffering that women experience in the lead up to making informed decisions about cosmetic surgery, but also in their heroism to take action and obtain surgery. Davis summarizes her case thus:

> My analysis is situated on the razor's edge between a feminist critique of the cosmetic surgery craze (along with the ideologies of feminine inferiority which sustain it) and an equally feminist desire to treat women as

agents who negotiate their bodies and their lives within the cultural and structural constraints of a gendered social order. This has meant exploring cosmetic surgery as one of the most pernicious expressions of the Western beauty culture without relegating women who have it to the position of 'cultural dope'. It has involved understanding how cosmetic surgery might be the best possible course of action for a particular women, while, at the same time, problematizing the situational constraints which make cosmetic surgery an option.[17]

Seeking to move away from the oppression/liberation model that renders women as 'cultural dopes', Davis develops an analytical approach that emphasizes the agency and autonomy of women in relation to cosmetic surgery. She writes of 'taking one's life in one's own hands', 'taking control' and 'getting one's life in hand'. How all this might apply to the case of a New York woman who wanted to have liposuction on her toes is not easy to see. But if Davis equates agency with action, in an attempt to show how women's participation in the beauty industry may be potentially liberating or subversive, she also runs the risk of reproducing some of the worst, voluntaristic clichés about cosmetic surgical culture. Thus, at times, her portrayal of the heroism of women who actually undergo surgery reads a little like the advertising sections of *Cosmopolitan* or *Vogue*.

There is also the question of whether cosmetic surgery is always consumerist or celebrity-inspired. For most people today, cosmetic surgery is increasingly equated with the rise of consumer culture, particularly as regards appearance, the remaking of the body, indeed life itself. Even so, many people would recognize that, while consumer and celebrity cultures may be a powerful influence on attitudes to cosmetic surgery, social attitudes and opinions are not ultimately reducible to such forces. That is to say, real-life cosmetic surgery involves a whole range of issues – from aesthetic concerns to medical and health matters to life-style considerations.

Yet for a host of exponents of the thesis of cosmetic surgery as pure (patriarchal) oppression, there can be no greater analytical naivety than confusing the makeover industries with the autonomous, self-legislating decisions of free individuals. For advocates of this standpoint, cosmetic surgical culture is overwhelmingly determined by the interplay of consumerism, celebrity and patriarchal culture. One of the most sophisticated recent studies of cosmetic surgery from this angle, Virginia L. Blum's *Flesh Wounds: The Culture of Cosmetic Surgery*, regards the consumption of alluring and enticing body images as foundational to cosmetic surgical culture itself. She writes:

> The greater popularity and increased normalization of plastic surgery as a bodily practice at the turn of the millennium are the results of a population of people who identify with two-dimensional images as our most permanent form of 'value'.[18]

Through a heady blend of feminist theory, psychoanalysis and cultural studies, Blum interrogates the psychic and subjective processes that render individuals 'addicted to surgery'. The argument, whilst involving sophisticated readings and applications of Freudian and Lacanian psychoanalysis, seems to be that a fundamental human ambivalence holds cosmetic surgical culture in check – at once reproducing, extending and cancelling itself. Drawing inspiration from the late French sociologist Jean Baudrillard's notion of *simulacra*, Blum concludes that

> the plastic surgery of the multitudes could be read not only as the culmination of the incursions of star culture but also its ultimate undoing . . . Just as the television watches us, perhaps we are now the models – or rather,

models of models, whose thoroughly internalised two-dimensionality functions as the ever-receding basis for 'human' performances.[19]

Radical feminist theory, though this time in a Foucault-ian rather than Lacanian vein, also informs Victoria Pitts-Taylor's *Surgery Junkies*. In an abstract treatment of the topic, Pitts-Taylor manages the unusual feat of 'following the insights of postmodern and poststructural social theory' in order to 'declare the truth of individual subjectivities' under-going cosmetic surgery, all the while remaining mostly unconcerned with the actual experience of people undergo-ing the surgeon's knife. Very little of the book gives any hint that cosmetic surgery involves anything other than a text-book application of Foucault's thesis of 'technologies of the self'. Pitts-Taylor's analysis then depends on a shift from liposuction to language as the centre of focus. 'I see the bodies of cosmetic surgery', writes Pitts-Taylor in high Foucaultian rhetoric,

> as sites of visibility where the self is exposed. That we speak so much about the self and see it on the body's surface are not because we have found the real truth of cosmetic surgery, but because we are moved to consider and find this truth in historically specific ways.[20]

This is far removed from the conventional wisdom as to why people desire, say, liposuction. Throughout the book, Pitts-Taylor's tone is not exactly that of a philosophy tutor-ial, but it's not that far off either. Towards the conclusion of *Surgery Junkies*, surprisingly and disarmingly, she provides 'an autoethnographic account' of her own cosmetic surgery: during the course of researching her book, Pitts-Taylor under-went rhinoplasty. But any reader expecting to get closer to the cut and thrust of cosmetic surgery will find disappoint-ment in store here, such is Pitts-Taylor's dry, academicist,

lecture-note style. This is perhaps most graphically illus-
trated by her following reflection on what prompted her
decision to undergo the surgeon's knife:

> I was initially motivated by a desire to put myself into the
> role of the patient, but I was also attracted to the idea that
> I could be more beautiful, my deep training in critiques
> of heteronormativity nothwithstanding.[21]

It would seem clear that, in this instance, philosophy and
cosmetic surgery don't mix.

At perhaps even higher levels of conceptual abstrac-
tion and political obscurantism, other critics have sought to
hunt down the all-inclusive definition, or determining cause,
of cosmetic surgical culture. In *Technologies of the Gendered
Body*, Anne Balsamo holds that cosmetic surgery is a practice through which 'women consciously act to make their
bodies mean something to themselves and to others'.[22] In
high semiotic mode, she contends that 'cosmetic surgery literally transforms the material body into a sign of culture'.[23]
When, however, is the body not a sign of culture? One can
only wonder how it is that the standard 'pre-cosmetic' body
(Balsam's 'material body') stands outside culture. Similarly,
consider Suzanne Fraser, who defines the field thus:

> As a machinic assemblage, cosmetic surgery combines
> discourses, people (both as recipients and as profession-
> als, such as doctors, lawyers, psychologists, advertising
> agents and scientists), equipment and locations (hospitals,
> clinics, courtrooms, etc.).[24]

It is not easy to see from this standpoint how the work of a
cosmetic surgeon differs from that of a prosthodontist or
brain surgeon.

Then there is the legion of 'insiders guides' to cosmetic
surgery. In *The Facelift Diaries*, an unintentionally humorous

35

guide by two psychoanalytic clinicians who had under-gone surgery, Jill Scharff and Jaedene Levy remark:

> Once a women knows you've had a facelift, she feels connected to you. Once she knows, she claims the right to examine your face openly and make comments. A facelift puts you out there, and asks you to look into yourself.[25]

Such pop psychology tells us very little, except that cosmetic surgery for the authors 'puts you out there' in a way apparently different from, say, Pilates, scuba-diving or stock-market trading. It is revealing that Scharff and Levy spend the bulk of the book documenting their every self-doubt, anxiety, bodily suffering and interpersonal strain with family, friends and patients. 'When we were young', they write,

> we were sure that there was something quite wonder-ful about seeing life experience etched in the lines of the face. As we got older we agreed that some people age beautifully but we found that we were not among them. Our faces were sending out the wrong messages about us.

Clearly, their profession, psychoanalysis, was of little assis-tance to Scharff and Levy in coming to terms with the 'wrong messages' emitted by their faces.

Alex Kuczynski's *Beauty Junkies*, by contrast, is a bracing encounter with cosmetic surgery written by someone at once inside and outside its culture. The author's insider status comes from her work as a *New York Times* journalist who has written extensively about cosmetic surgical culture and its pathologies; yet, as a recovering Botox addict and beauty junkie, she develops a stinging, ironic social critique. Kuczyn-ski's gripping exploration of all things cosmetic is relayed primarily through lively anecdotes – ranging from the Manhattan 'foot face-lift' specialist offering microdermabrasion for toes and feet to the fat transfer doctor providing for the surgical reassignment of fat from the bottom to the face for New York ladies who lunch. Extreme makeovers for Kuczynski are part and parcel of the American lifestyle. 'The notion that we can enhance our looks', writes Kuczynski,

> is terrifically appealing to insecure Americans. And there are in fact more reasons cropping up to contribute to our growing self-loathing: we're getting fatter and older and more unhealthy by the minute. A wealth of mini-industries and leisure activities has sprung up around the cosmetic surgery industry, dictating everything from what we read to what we watch to how we think.[26]

It is the interweaving of makeover industries and cosmetic surgical culture that interests Kuczynski, although the journalistic orientation of her book precludes analysis of the new interpenetration of cosmetics and commerce. Nevertheless, she does understand that the culture of cosmetic surgery is toxic. Reflecting on her own Restylane disaster, which left her temporarily with nightmare inflatable lips, she writes:

> trying to remain beautiful and stay young looking is, paradoxically, a young person's game. No matter how many antioxidant vitamins we swallow or Botox shots we get, we live in a constant state of disintegration. In an era in which we aspire to the constant upgrade – we upgrade our houses, spouses, cars, breasts – we inhabit physical machines that are insistently downgrading us all the time.[27]

That cosmetic surgery has been debated in both highly abstract and sensationalist forms should come as no surprise.

But there have also been less eye-catching, very technical kinds of discussion over cosmetic surgery and its consequences. In 2007, during the course of researching this book, I attended a summer meeting of academics, bioethicists and policy makers from the European Union at the University of Vienna. Staying at the grand Hotel Astoria near the well-known Karntnerstrasse, just a few steps from the famous Vienna State Opera, my initial impression was that the rich cultural history of the city appeared somewhat at odds with the challenges of biomedicine and the new technologies that the conference delegates had come together to debate.

The conference was titled 'Engineering European Bodies', and was part of a broader EU project on European governance and bioethics. I had, mistakenly as it happens, assumed that the conference would be largely an exercise in critique linking medicine, technology and society. I had imagined that participants would seek to place cosmetic surgery within the institutional changes that have marked our time: new technologies, globalization and accelerating individualism. But I was wrong. Few of the people at the conference appeared remotely concerned with the social and political consequences of cosmetic surgical culture. Rather, this was a gathering of technical specialists and policy wonks concerned with mapping common governance regulations for biomedical technologies and their reshaping of bodies and identities throughout the European Union. In effect, the conference reflected the instrumental imperatives that have so powerfully shaped cosmetic surgical culture across Europe. Yet what was on offer was, by and large, an analysis of bodies strangely bloodless, of identities peculiarly devoid of emotion. These specialists and policy experts were not at the conference to question and critique cosmetic surgical culture; they were there to work out how to make it *function* more efficiently. As I sat listening to presentations with such titles as 'Translating Experience into Biomedical

Assemblages', 'Moving Bioethics beyond Ethics' and 'Transhumanist Challenges to Virtue Ethics', I realized that my fellow delegates were the last people one would consult in order to learn about the personal and emotional challenges individuals face when contemplating cosmetic surgery.

One presenter who did spark my curiosity, however, was Michael Zichy from the Ludwig-Maximilian University in Munich. Zichy's interest is in the relation between surgical enhancement and ethics, biotechnological bodily sculpting and moral issues about identity. According to Zichy, surgical enhancement through biotechnological means raises fundamental ethical questions about who we are and who we want to be. 'The technical term "enhancement"', says Zichy, 'serves as a focal point for human dreams, hopes, promises and fears.'[28] Having reviewed scientific, technical and public discourses of surgical enhancement in the light of shared European values, Zichy concludes that there are four main approaches, images or assumptions evident in all statements and opinions. These consist of (1), a scientific, progress-focused ideology that locates cosmetic surgical enhancement in terms of a moral need for individual or bodily transformation; (2) a liberalistic approach with a thin conception of identity, one that constructs enhancement in terms of life options; (3) a humanistic approach that values enhancement to the extent that this promotes equality among people; and (4) an essentialist approach that rejects cosmetic surgical enhancement on the grounds that 'human nature' should not be interfered with or altered. Alternatively, these approaches might be redescribed as core ideologies proscribing why one *should, could, might* or *shouldn't* undertake cosmetic surgical enhancement of the body.

Such analytical categories might be profitably deployed to grasp the broader public debate over cosmetic surgery in recent years. To the extent that we have witnessed the emergence of such a debate, and this has been very patchy across contemporary societies, the standard argument has tended to divide between those who are pro-choice and those who claim cosmetic surgical culture is coterminous with the creation of new personal vulnerabilities on a societal level. For those who defend cosmetic surgery, especially plastic surgeons and the professional associations, it is consumer choice that is particularly valued in this context, which may be the reason this argument has gained such a sympathetic public hearing. Cosmetic surgery and the related makeover industries, it is claimed, provide individuals with opportunities to negotiate or acquire a unique identity based on individual self-choice. And to the extent that change is considered desirable in itself, which it is for such professional advocates of perpetual plasticity, cosmetic surgery is said to promote advancements in personal autonomy, which in itself is a public good. This pro-choice standpoint would appear to reduce to the simplistic viewpoint that as long as people make the right decisions – from the moisturizer one puts on in the morning to the surgical enhancements one undertakes from time to time – all in life will work out fine. From this angle, and invoking Zichy's scheme, cosmetic surgery is a practice one certainly might or could undertake, and possibly should. On the other hand, critics of cosmetic surgical culture have expressed alarm at the sheer emotional cost, as well as potential social dislocation, arising from such pre-packaged refashionings of the body. On this view, there may well be solid reasons to 'personalize' identity in line with the myriad of cultural styles now on offer within the marketplace, but to re-sculpt the body completely is a step too far. For such critics, cosmetic surgical culture is shot through with extreme narcissism, adolescent to its core, generative of new personal vulnerabilities and the instigator of a dangerous cultural addiction. It is, to be sure, a practice one *shouldn't* undertake (or, this is so reading such criticism through the lens of Zichy's scheme).

These broadly evaluative terms 'for' and 'against' pervade most aspects of public and academic discussions of cosmetic and plastic surgery. But one of the paradoxes of such narrow framing of this debate, in my view, is that deeper social and institutional forces governing the production of cosmetic surgical culture remain widely ignored. My quarrel with academics and public intellectuals pronouncing on the gains and losses of cosmetic surgery is not whether it leads to the corrosion of identity or advances a better future; attitudes, orientations and beliefs about self-reinvention have indeed changed in recent times, and it may not be sociologically possible (or even desirable) to attempt a cost / benefit analysis of such social trends. My argument is that the new individualism of instant change promoted by cosmetic surgical culture is shaped by, and is reshaping, wider institutional changes associated with globalization. The aim of this book is not simply to discuss in a serious fashion a social issue that is regularly trivialized, but to interrogate the social forces contributing to the escalation of cosmetic surgical culture more generally.

Why, as a society, are we increasingly held in thrall to cosmetic surgical culture? And what drives people to contemplate extreme reinvention by undergoing the surgeon's knife? Throughout this book I will seek to answer these central questions.

To both questions there is a marvellously appealing answer, usually given by the media but also increasingly by academics. It comes down to two words: celebrity culture. The explosion of celebrity culture in these early years of the twenty-first century, it is widely argued, is intimately interwoven with the spread of new technologies for making private life a public spectacle. In such circumstances, the dissemination of new technologies – from DVDs and satellite television to mobile phones and camcorders – has given audiences unprecedented opportunities to view, examine and scrutinize their favourite celebrities at close proximity. Consequently, as media technologies have increasingly penetrated the fabric of daily life, celebrities have reacted by continually updating and changing their appearance, transforming their image and, in particular, seeking artificially enhanced beauty.

Celebrity culture, no doubt, does help to explain some aspects of the widespread explosion of interest in cosmetic surgery. It is surely the case, for example, that today media and public scrutiny of celebrity bodies is more intense than ever before. The most trivial lifestyle routines of the rich and famous – from a star's beauty routine to how often they work out at the gym – are chronicled by the media in painstaking detail. The odd academic study that does consider media culture today usually blames celebrity for reshaping public attitudes about identity, self-reinvention and the body. But this explanation is remarkably simplistic, assuming as it does that celebrity culture is catapulted into our daily lives from outer space. It assumes that the vast majority of people are drawn to artificially enhanced beauty simply as a result of 'external' forces (namely, the media), and thus downgrades the deeper emotional and societal factors propelling people into a more active engagement with self-reinvention. Such dismissal of the restructuring of relations between public and private life is common. Yet celebrities do more than merely reflect technological power; they also embody, enact and represent technology. In a world of continuous global media, in which artificially enhanced beauty is very desirable, celebrity experimentations with cosmetic surgery capture the breathtaking changes now occurring within society as regards the open-ended relation between identity and the body, as well as the increasing centrality of self-reinvention as part of life. Demi Moore, Pamela Anderson, Dannii Minogue, Melanie Griffith and Courtney Love are representatives of the celebrity-led plastic surgery revolution.

Any analysis of the rise of cosmetic surgery that ignored celebrity culture would be gravely insufficient, and in the following chapter I shall turn to a range of new social trends to do with self-reinvention, the mass media and celebrity. That said, there are good reasons to suppose that what I shall call the celebrity culture thesis cannot alone explain the impacts that cosmetic surgery and the makeover industries are having on our lives today. For one thing, the idea that all of us are held in thrall to a culture of Botox and bling is surely misplaced. It is certainly the case that magazines such as *People* and *Who Weekly*, as well as television programmes such as *Entertainment Tonight* and *E News*, document the surgical enhancements and cosmetic addictions of celebrities the world over, or at least the 'world' as defined in the image of American popular culture. But this does not mean that all individuals want to remake themselves with the reinvention rapidity of Posh and Becks, Madonna or Kylie Minogue.

Another popular explanation focuses on consumerism. To a greater or lesser degree, we are all caught up – so the argument goes – in the consumption, or purchase, of desired identities, bodies and artificially framed styles of life. We devour images of 'the good life'. We opt for one of the lifestyles available from standardized, packaged consumption. We live for the consumption of ever-novel goods, services and lifestyles. Much of the world as we know it is what we know through shopping. Old-style shopping for 'things' gives way to the consumption of our emotions, our experiences and our lifestyles. The pursuit of personal autonomy or self-definition, for example, is seemingly impossible without consumption of 'identity commodities' – the appointment with a therapist, the purchase of a self-help book, the daily trip to the gym.

Cosmetic surgical culture is one area of life where such commodifying of consumption plays itself out with a vengeance. From dermal fillers to breast augmentation, advertisers seek to reorder existing behaviour patterns around the purchase of enhanced body parts. This involves a lifting of the consumer-orientated mentality to the second power, such that people are, literally, purchasing themselves. In 2007 journalist Natasha Singer, from the *New York Times*, noted a dramatic rise in the numbers of people financing cosmetic surgery with loans and credit cards, a powerful indication of the impact of commodification in itself. Singer linked cosmetic surgery and commodification as follows:

> Doctors around the country are noting a democratization of cosmetic medicine, a redefinition of it as a coveted yet attainable luxury purchase, on par with products like Louis Vuitton handbags or flat-screen televisions. The medical industry has responded by marketing plastic surgery as if it were an appliance or other big-ticket consumer product: a commodity to be financed with credit cards and loans . . . One of the most vivid illustrations of this economic reality is the rise of finance companies offering middle-income patients easy access to credit to pay for their surgeries. Patients throughout the country find brochures in their doctor's office with slogans like 'Get the Cosmetic Procedure You Want — Today!' from established financing companies like Capital One and CareCredit, a unit of GE Money.[29]

Commodification is in some ways even more insidious than this account indicates. For not only are people increasingly prepared to go into debt to finance their desires for flatter stomachs, bigger breasts and younger-looking faces, but many are also turning to monthly instalment plans that finance such body procedures for as little as a few dollars a month. The commodification of 'enhanced body parts' is today factored into people's budgets, and on a daily, weekly or monthly reckoning.

In addition to examining explanations that focus on celebrity culture and consumer industries for the dramatic rise in cosmetic surgery today, *Making the Cut* develops a new account of cosmetic surgical culture and its relation to individuals. Transformations in the new economy and in self-identity, I want to propose, are increasingly becoming intermeshed in conditions of advanced globalization. Changes in the institutional dimensions of organizational life, particularly in communications, service and high-finance sectors of the economy, are more and more tied to transformations in both working and personal life. In such circumstances, the fast-paced, techy culture of globalization is unleashing a new paradigm of self-making in which individuals are required to pick themselves up by their bootstraps and get on with the tasks, and daily, of reinventing, restructuring, remoulding and resculpting the self. This new paradigm, as I will argue at length in this book, has resulted in the reinvention craze sweeping contemporary societies – and it is nowhere better dramatized than in cosmetic surgical culture. This paradigm, advanced by business leaders, politicians, personal trainers and therapy gurus, emphasizes that flexible and ceaseless reinvention is the only adequate personal response to life in a globalizing world. It is a paradigm that pervades the mission statement of countless makeover service providers: personal trainers, spas, gyms, weight-loss and detox centres, cosmetic dentists and plastic surgeons all chasing the money that people will spend to realize their reinvention ideal.

Various factors, in conditions of advanced globalization, directly influence why individuals turn to the 'reinvention craze', as well as more specifically contemplate undergoing the plastic surgeon's knife in order to obtain a career edge. I do not claim in the pages that follow that cosmetic surgical culture is wholly shaped or determined by recent changes in the global economy. But the new economy has ushered into existence changes of enormous magnitude, and in such a world people are under intense pressure to keep pace with the sheer speed of change. Seemingly secure jobs are wiped out literally overnight. Technology becomes obsolete almost as soon as it is released. Multinational corporations move their operations from country to country in search of the best profit margin. Women and men clamber frenetically to obtain new skills or be discarded on the scrapheap. In this new economy of short-term contracts, endless downsizings, just-in-time deliveries and multiple careers, one reason for self-reinvention through cosmetic surgery is to demonstrate a personal readiness for change, flexibility and adaptability.

The reinvention craze paradigm extends beyond the core of the self to the body, that distracting reminder of mortality in a world where disposability has been elevated over durability, plasticity over permanence. The culture of speed and short-termism promoted by the global electronic economy, I shall argue in subsequent chapters, introduces fundamental anxieties and insecurities that are increasingly resolved by individuals at the level of the body. Bodies today are pumped, pummelled, plucked, suctioned, stitched, shrunk and surgically augmented at an astonishing rate. It is not my argument that the cosmetic redesign of the body arises because of the appearance of completely novel anxieties. Previous ages have been plagued by anxiety too, and certainly insecurities pertaining to employment and career prospects are hardly new.[30] But the method of coping with, and reacting to, anxieties stemming from the new paradigm of self-making in our global age is quite different from previous times. In contrast to the factory-conditioned certainties and bureaucratic rigidities of yesterday's work world, in which personal insecurities 'locked in' tightly with the organizational settings of economic life, today's new corporatism is a world in which individuals are increasingly left to their own devices as regards their working life and its future prospects. This is a societal change that creates considerable scope for personal opportunities, but it is also one that involves severe stresses and emotional costs. Today's faith in flexibility, plasticity and incessant reinvention throughout the corporate world means that employees are judged less and less on previous achievements, on their records. Rather, people are assessed, and ever more so, on their willingness to embrace change, their adaptability for personal makeover. In such circumstances, anxiety becomes free-floating, *detached* from organizational life. Consequently, anxiety rounds back upon the self. In such circumstances, many feel an increased pressure to improve, transform, alter and reinvent themselves. Cosmetic surgical culture arises in this social space, in response to such ambient fears.

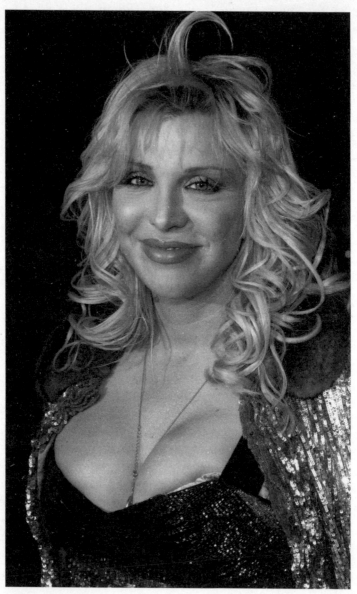

Courtney Love, 2006.

Chapter 2

Celebrity Obsession: Fame, Fortune and Faking It

In May 2007 the Australian media noted a 70 per cent rise in cosmetic operation lawsuits in the wake of a major surgery fallout. Widespread media reporting in newspapers, magazines, radio and television documented more than AUS$4 million worth of claims against plastic and cosmetic surgeons, particularly cosmetic medical practitioners. From botched breast augmentations to failed face-lifts, the scientific advancement, innovation and progress associated with the culture of nip and tuck were momentarily called into question by news of the skyrocketing number of negligence claims against cosmetic practitioners.

Central to this surgery fallout was the story of Kerry Mullins. A married mother of five children living in Melbourne, Mullins had booked an appointment with one of the city's leading plastic surgeons following the birth of her last child. In consultation with her surgeon concerning her desire to undergo a 'total makeover', Mullins was advised to have a 'mum's makeover' – the cost of which was estimated in excess of $25,000. As designed for Mullins, this consisted of a breast lift, tummy tuck and full liposuction – including her chin, underarms and inner thighs. The prospect of breast implants, it seems, particularly enticed Mullins: such a breast lift would return to her a pre-baby body. Commenting on the promises made by her surgeon, Mullins later commented: 'he said he would sew my abs back together so it looked like I never had babies and the tummy tuck would only leave a 10 cm c-section scar'.[1]

There was just one stumbling block, or so it then seemed: the $25,000 price tag for the 'mum's makeover'. The costs of family living, especially in the wake of the newly arrived fifth child, were already soaring – and the Mullins didn't have the required cash reserves to go ahead with such custom-made surgery. Desperate to find a solution, they mortgaged a family home in the UK to fund Kerry's makeover.

Millions of cosmetic procedures are performed the world over each year and most are deemed cosmetically successful. Not so, however, Kerry Mullins's cosmetic alteration. Arriving at one of Melbourne's leading private hospitals in early 2006, Mullins underwent the surgeon's knife in order to have several areas of her body treated during one procedure. Early indications of difficulty arose when she awoke in pain after the operation, reporting discomfort in her right breast. Some hours later, this pain intensified; subsequently, there was discolouring of the tissue of her breast. She was in turn discharged from the hospital. Sometime later she returned to a surgery day clinic to receive treatment for a 'breast infection'. In time the pain developed into agony, and Mullins returned to hospital to have her infected breast splayed open and cleaned. The dramatic fallout for the surgical profession came, however, when it was reported that Mullins's dream of a makeover came at the cost of leaving her without a breast at all.

Mullins's makeover dream did not originate in a social vacuum. For like countless women and men living in the polished, expensive cities of the West, her daily reality was powerfully influenced by media stories about people undergoing extreme self-reinvention. Of crucial significance to this reinvention currency has been the explosion of interest in reality TV and makeover programmes. Kerry Mullins's makeover hell had its roots in such extreme makeover TV shows, and by implication the cultural landscape of fame and surgically enhanced celebrity bodies.

The conduit of celebrity arises from massive institutional changes throughout the West, involving a wholesale shift from industrial manufacture to a post-industrial economy orientated to the finance, service and communications sectors. As the economy becomes cultural, ever more dependent on media, image and public relations, so personal identity comes under the spotlight and open to revision. The new economy, in which the globalization of media looms large, celebrates both technological culture and the power of new technologies to reshape the links between society, the body and the self. The current cultural obsession with artificially enhanced beauty is reflective of this, and nowhere more so than in the attention that popular culture lavishes upon celebrity. The relentless media scrutiny of celebrity bodies and their possible surgical transformations runs all the way from paparazzi and gossip magazines to entertainment news and high-definition television to awfulplasticsurgery.com and YouTube. From filler injections to neck lifts, the augmented faces and bodies of celebrities are monitored continuously by popular culture and the wider society. And it is much of this heady cosmetic brew that spreads, in turn, throughout everyday life – as the mesmerizing artificial beauty of celebrities inspires people to turn to cosmetic surgical culture.

Extreme makeover TV shows are the latest form in and through which celebrity culture infiltrates daily life. What's striking about many of these programmes is not only their continual referencing to cosmetic surgical culture, but how they normalize cosmetic surgery in the stories they document. Programmes such as American network ABC's *Extreme Makeover* and the UK Channel 4's *10 Years Younger*, which uses cosmetic procedures to 'redesign' women, as well as various cable offerings including *Cosmetic Surgery*

Live, *The Swan* and MTV's *I Want a Famous Face*, are creating a new emotional climate in which people are increasingly seduced by drastic head-to-toe surgery. Advanced plastic surgery, high-tech cosmetic enhancements to the body, cosmetic dentistry and novel exercise and diet regimes are routinely used in such programmes to enhance beauty artificially, to re-sculpt the body and to restructure the self.

The Swan, one of the most successful American makeover shows, illustrates the way in which surgical enhancements of the body are becoming symbolically equated with the re-creation of self-identity at a broad cultural and societal level. Throughout countless episodes, *The Swan* seeks to document the authenticity of its remaking of identities by focusing on 'before' and 'after' body shots of its participants. The penultimate detailing of the programme's remaking of bodies comes in a section known as 'The Reveal'. Here women who have undergone intensive plastic surgery and related cosmetic procedures are 'unveiled' in front of a live audience – usually comprising friends and family as well as the TV hosts. At this point, the 'contestant' seeks to 'read' the expression of the faces all around her as an indication of the level of self-transformation that has been performed on her; the 'contestant' is thus presented as not having seen for herself the final results of her cosmetic surgery. As David Lyle, producer of *The Swan*, comments: 'I defy you not to watch that moment when the curtain goes back, and the person sees what's happened to them.' Separating contestants off from any monitoring or self-knowledge of their personal makeover until the end of the programme is thus an essential ingredient of *The Swan*, as if to extend at the level of fantasy the power that new cosmetic technologies have over and above individuals. For 'the reveal', as Lyle aptly puts it, 'is almost the pornographic shot. Let's face it – slapping a new coat of paint on is not as dramatic as having someone carve your face off.'

In linking 'the reveal' and 'the pornographic shot', Lyle's thinking here picks up on broader connections between cosmetic surgery culture on the one hand and pornography on the other. For some critics, this link can be discerned in the ways that cosmetic surgical culture challenges received ideas regarding the limits of identity and the body, perhaps in a fashion akin to how pornography destabilizes cultural taboos regarding sexuality. Channel 5's *Cosmetic Surgery Live* in the UK, for example, has shown graphic images of extreme surgical requests the world over – including a man who consulted a cosmetic practitioner to have his anus bleached. Sometimes the social messages and cultural images surrounding surgical culture are a little more subtle, though most are still highly influenced by the twin forces of advanced capitalism and the soft-porn images of celebrity culture.

In the past few years, reality makeover TV shows have redefined and extended the range of 'body parts' potentially subject to the interventions of surgical culture. From America's *Extreme Makeover* to Poland's *Make Me Beautiful*, women (and sometimes men) have willingly had cosmetic and surgical work performed on their lips, noses, chins, eyes, cheeks, breasts, thighs and bottoms. To this extent, reality makeover TV shows are at one with the reduction of women's bodies to various 'part-objects'.[2] What's interesting about such programmes, in contrast to the short-term, instant gratification promoted by the global porn industry, is how the *narrative* of extreme reinvention is extended across episodes. The narrative structure of such programmes is now familiar, ranging as it does from the identification of 'bodily defects', and associated degrees of personal unhappiness resulting from such deficiencies, to the multiple procedures available for the correction and enhancement and on to the final 'reveal'. It is this reality TV narrative of possibilities for instant self-reinvention that runs through celebrity culture and increasingly all the way down to societal attitudes.

In his magisterial study of the history of fame, *The Frenzy of Renown*, Leo Braudy traces the many different ways in which representations of the famous have been disseminated.[3] From traditional societies in which gods, priests and saints were famous through to the era of Hollywood and its invention of film stars, different societies and cultures have developed particular methods for the dissemination of information about public figures. Braudy focuses especially on how fame is dependant on media dissemination, and highlights how the urge to fame is increasingly personalized with the advent of mass communications and popular culture. He underscores, for example, the complex ways in which personal authenticity, artistic originality and individual creativity have shaped, and have been shaped by, forms of public attention. From Laurence Olivier's dramatic talents to Rudolf Nureyev's ballet grace, from Groucho Marx's comic genius to John Lennon's pop music brilliance: the true artist of the modernist era was one who distinguished themselves through the expression of their personal gifts, their 'inner genius', lifting them out from the surrounds of the wider society.

By contrast, today's globalized world of new information technologies and media transformations turns both the production and reception of fame upside down. We have witnessed in recent years a large-scale shift from Hollywood definitions of fame to multi-media-driven forms of public recognition. This new field of 'publicness' signals a general transformation from 'fame' to 'celebrity'. This has involved a very broad change from narrow, elite definitions of public renown to more open, inclusive understandings. This *democratization of public renown* has gone hand in hand with the rise of celebrity culture. Celebrity today hinges increasingly on the capacity of the celebrated to create a distance (however minimal) from what originally brought them to public notice, thereby opening a media space from which to project their celebrity in novel and innovative ways. In a sense, celebrity might be described as fame emptied of content, or artistry. What is striking is not simply how celebrities transform and reinvent their identities, but how many of them embrace and indeed celebrate a culture of inauthenticity. If originality and authenticity were the hallmarks of traditional notions of fame, then parody, pastiche and above all sudden transformations in a star's identity are the crucial indicators of contemporary celebrity.

Perhaps more than any other area of instant self-transformation, celebrity culture is noted for the attention it lavishes on plastic surgery and related cosmetic procedures. Today the surgical enhancement, remoulding and tightening of celebrity bodies borders on a public obsession – as any casual glance of popular magazines or infotainment TV programmes will confirm. From Dolly Parton to Heidi Klum, Sylvester Stallone to Jennifer Aniston, Courtney Love to Paris Hilton, Mickey Rourke to Michael Douglas, the array of speculation regarding artificially enhanced celebrity bodies is testament to the high visibility of cosmetic surgical culture. And not only are celebrities increasingly willing (perhaps required?) to undergo the surgeon's knife; many are also willing to acknowledge, and even discuss, their experiments with surgery in the media and wider public sphere.

One of the best examples of such an embracement of cosmetic surgery by contemporary celebrity culture is the career of Pamela Anderson. Breast implants initially helped land Anderson a role in the globally watched TV programme *Baywatch*, establishing the buxom blonde as one of the most recognized figures of popular culture. As Anderson commented in an interview, 'my implants are definitely one of my biggest assets. They increase my femininity and make me more noticeable.'[4] Her comment is remarkably explicit in drawing a direct connection between enhanced breast size / enhanced femininity on the one hand, and heightened levels of public attention on the other. Anderson's overtly plastic appearance was not without its problems, however, including media speculation of medical issues associated with her surgery. In time, she had the implants reduced. 'I'm a petite person who no longer feels right as a large-breasted Dolly Parton', she explained. Anderson's breast downsizing did not last for long, however. For the 2002 Academy Awards, she arrived to display what various commentators called 'new super implants'.

If Pamela Anderson is a classic example of the intricate connections between contemporary celebrity transform-ations and the culture of nip and tuck, then American singer Cher raises this equation to the second power. Widely hailed in the media as 'the plastic surgery poster girl', Cher underwent the surgeon's knife with a breast implant procedure, rhinoplasty and laser surgery for the removal of her many tattoos. Other media speculation also suggests that she has undergone procedures for cheek im-plants, tummy tucks, butt-lifts and liposuction. Respond-ing to media questioning about her reasons for having breast implants, she commented: 'Oh, because they got so much bigger after Chastity was born, and I couldn't bear to see them deflate.'[5] Neither, it seems could her fans; nor the media, producing as they did endless stories document-ing the radical remoulding of her breasts.

Celebrity, I am suggesting, is becoming increasingly syn-onymous with self-reinvention, and nowhere is this more evident than famous people experimenting with artifi-cially enhanced beauty as a means of demonstrating their celebrity status. Increasingly, celebrities are implanting and injecting, suturing and (lipo)suctioning, all in the quest for artificial beauty. Celebrity-inspired self-transformation is, in broader social terms, a condensation of how many indi-viduals now experience and define their lives as fluid, multiple, even liquid. The new social paradigm of instant self-reinvention fuels such thinking, and the possibilities opened up by celebrity-led surgical culture provides a vivid

– if at times extreme – indication of such crucial changes between self and society. At least, that is the proposition I now want to explore, considering cosmetic surgical culture specifically in terms of a transfer from celebrity to fandom.

Consider, for example, the story of Sha, a nineteen-year-old contestant from Texas who appeared on the MTV reality programme *I Want a Famous Face*. Focused on a career in modelling, and with an appearance in the 'college edition' of *Playboy* already to her name, Sha applied as a contestant to *I Want a Famous Face* on the grounds that she wanted to *look* more like Pamela Anderson. The programme's expert panel concluded that Sha's dream was not impossible for the Texan beauty, but advised that in order to achieve her ideal it would be necessary for her to undergo a personal makeover. Their recommendation consisted of a breast implant procedure, lip implants and liposuction under her chin. The injecting of filler fluids and implanting, it was said, would do wonders for Sha's post-surgical modelling career. As it happens, Sha proved a model contestant. An avid fan of celebrity culture, attuned to the demands of cosmetic surgery, with seemingly little personal anxiety or worry about her course of action, Sha responded positively to the panel's recommendations. In a candid admission on the MTV website concerning the possibilities and the pain that cosmetic surgery involved for her, Sha's 'Post-op Interview' unfolds in the following fashion:

> MTV: Are you pleased with the results of your surgery?
> SHA: Yes.
> MTV: Was it worth it? Why or why not?
> SHA: It was worth it because I love all the attention I have gotten and it has made me feel so much better about myself.
> MTV: What was the biggest post-surgery surprise?
> SHA: The pain and how much it really did hurt.

MTV: Was it painful?

SHA: Hell ya![6]

The remainder of the interview is equally theatrical. Sha talks of her hopes for a lucrative post-surgical modelling career. Yet the glaring contradiction between an improved sense of professional self-worth on the one hand and the pain of plastic surgery on the other remains unexplored. Why this shift from the acute pain of surgery to feeling 'so much better' about herself? Is the feeling of self-improvement connected, in some way, to the reality of pain? This is nowhere considered by Sha or her interviewees on the MTV website. Instead, just various post-surgery pictures are posted, as well as her poses for *Playboy*.

The realm of fans following after the image of celebrity culture regularly involves such high levels of denial or displacement. This is especially the case as regards the denial of bodily pain resulting from cosmetic surgery undertaken in the footsteps of the famous. In a recent study of the growing acceptance and approval of cosmetic surgery among Americans, sociologist Abigail Brooks reports on portrayals of the body in pain that are all but cancelled out through narratives of scientific progress, technological innovation, self-improvement or mental and physical health.[7] Brooks offers, amongst other examples, that of Patricia Heaton – star of the TV show *Everyone Loves Raymond* – and her experience of cosmetic surgery. Citing an interview in *People*, Heaton reflected:

I got to take Perocet, Valium, and Ambien all at the same time! That's right! Who knew? It was as if cutting me open, creating a new belly button and scraping seven years of scar tissue never happened.

Like Sha's narrative, Heaton's reflections mix the good and bad, the gains and losses – but this time with a humour that minimizes the side effects of cosmetic surgery. Whatever the implied pain issuing from cosmetic surgery, and hence Heaton's pleasure in recounting her heavy sedation, the experience itself is recalibrated through ironic humour. The suggestion, then, is that undergoing the surgeon's knife requires considerable courage or virtue. On a sociological level, Brooks finds that such narratives serve to *normalize* cosmetic surgery in ways that fracture established connections between self and body. As Brooks concludes: 'An aspect of bodily knowledge, wherein pain and bleeding are respected as meaningful, informative signals, recedes and an interventionist – receptive side effect – tolerant understanding of the body takes its place.'[8]

Popular media culture is today dominated by instant identity makeover television shows, celebrity confessions delivered on therapy-inspired daytime chat programmes and an extraordinary fascination with the artificial beauty enhancements of the rich and famous. Viewers of, and participants in, celebrity culture move in a world that is sometimes loosely called postmodern – by which is meant that our televisual world portrays a celebrity reality that is doubtfully real. Media coverage of celebrity events is captivating because it blurs traditional distinctions between fact and fiction, transporting the viewer to what the late French sociologist Jean Baudrillard termed 'hyperreality'. But there are aspects of current celebrity transformations, particularly as regards surgical culture, that are postmodern in a more specific sense too. Twenty-first-century media culture is increasingly a self-enclosed terrain in which what matters is not so much the portrayal of lives or reality in a linear timeframe, but how the continually reinvented self and its artificial augmentation is presented in the here and now. This has involved a telescoping downwards from the celebrated personality to celebrity bodies. Put succinctly, we have now entered a culture obsessed with the *body parts* of celebrities. Moreover, this cultural trend, in turn, depends on a kind of thinking involving (following the post-Freudian psychoanalyst Melanie Klein) splitting, denial and paranoia – of which more shortly.

In 2001 BBC News reported findings from a UK survey investigating women's attitudes to their bodies. Titled 'Most Women Want Plastic Surgery', the BBC noted that more than two-thirds of the 3,000 women questioned for the survey said that they would undergo plastic surgery to achieve the perfect celebrity look.[9] The ideal woman that emerged from the survey was an assemblage of various celebrity body parts. From those surveyed, the perfect female body comprised Liz Hurley's bust, Elle Macpherson's legs, Jennifer Lopez's bottom, Catherine Zeta-Jones's face and Jennifer Aniston's hair.

Several years later, in January 2004, *The Independent* in the UK presented its own findings on the most requested body parts. Presented in table form, this survey underscores even more graphically the cultural trend towards part-object thinking in contemporary culture.

BODY PART	WOMEN	MEN
Nose	Nicole Kidman	Ben Affleck
	Reese Witherspoon	Edward Burns
	Diane Lane	Jude Law
Hair	Jennifer Aniston	Richard Gere
	Debra Messing	Hugh Grant
	Sarah Jessica Parker	Pierce Brosnan
Eyes	Halle Berry	Brad Pitt
	J-Lo	Ralph Fiennes
	Cameron Diaz	
Lips	Liv Tyler	Brad Pitt

	Uma Thurman	Matt Damon
	Renée Zellweger	Benicio Del Toro
Jaw-line* / *Chin*	Salma Hayek	Johnny Depp*
	Julianne Moore	Matthew McConaughey*
	Kim Cattrall	Russell Crowe
		Kiefer Sutherland
		Matt LeBlanc
Cheeks	J-Lo	Leonardo DiCaprio
	Halle Berry	John Corbett
	Jennifer Garner	George Clooney
Sculpting	Angelina Jolie	Tom Cruise
	Britney Spears	Benjamin Bratt
	J-Lo	Matt Damon
Skin	Michelle Pfeiffer	Ethan Hawke
	Gwyneth Paltrow	Hayden Christensen
	Sandra Bullock	Ryan Phillippe

In early 2007 the Hollywood siren Angelina Jolie was voted the 'Sexiest Ever Sex Symbol' in a UK television poll.[10] Beating off some formidable competition from Marilyn Monroe, Beyoncé Knowles and Kylie Minogue, not to mention Elvis Presley and Johnny Depp, Jolie won female celebrity with the sexiest body and the celeb-style that was the sexiest 'ever'. Meanwhile, in Manhattan, Jolie was being celebrated less for her sex appeal than for her commitments to social justice. Appointed to the prestigious US Council on Foreign Relations, Jolie joined other council members, including Condoleezza Rice, Henry Kissinger and Alan Greenspan, to take part in deliberations on the changing nature of national-state power in world affairs. Of vital importance to Jolie's elevation to this policy forum was perhaps less her celebrity status than her work as a

United Nations goodwill ambassador, from which she has campaigned for the rights of refugees, AIDS orphans and disaster victims.

It might well be because of these contradictory images, these split representations of celebrity, that Angelina Jolie is the person more and more women want to transform themselves into. Or, put more accurately, there are aspects of Jolie's image that women want to copy. The part-objects they want copied are her exaggerated, almost cartoon-like lips, eyes and cheekbones. According to UCLA academic and dermatologist Professor Ava Shamban, 'Angelina Jolie, with her exquisite looks, is the current gold standard of beauty in the United States and in the West in general right now.'[11] Moreover, the prevalence of such images will remain deeply anchored in Western culture for the foreseeable future. As Shamban adds, 'That's not about to change. The exotic look, like actresses Halle Berry and Penelope Cruz, is here to stay, and Angelina is the ultimate embodiment of that.'

There can be little doubt that Shamban is well placed to comment on the number of American women wanting a nip and tuck in the image of Angelina Jolie. A minor celebrity specialist herself, Shamban frequently appears on makeover programmes such as *Extreme Reinvention*, as well as in glossy magazines including *Vogue*, *Cosmopolitan* and *Tatler*. And as she notes, if the exotic celebrity image of Jolie is of particular appeal to Americans, it also strikes a chord throughout the West in general. Considering the links between the culture of celebrity and cosmetic surgical culture, Michael Zacharia, President of the Australian College of Cosmetic Surgery, comments: 'It's common to hear people say "I want lips or cheekbones like Angelina Jolie's".'

How is it that celebrity bodies become crucial sites of identification, imitation and desire – to such an extent that ordinary people are prepared to undergo the surgeon's knife? What is it that leads people to say, 'Make me look like her'? A sceptic might say, it all comes down to sex. And there may be some truth to this. After all, what else might provoke a woman to spend considerable resources, and to endure the often excruciating pain of surgery, outside the search for a kind of beauty that is the 'sexiest ever'. And, yet, more complex forces are at work here – involving sexuality certainly, but also the power of emotions, the aesthetic, and shifting boundaries between private and public life.

Unprecedented levels of interest in the lives, loves and scandals of celebrities, and particularly fascination with their cosmetic secrets and surgeries, have been widely viewed as a central driving force of cosmetic surgical culture. Many practitioners and surgeries report that when patients decide to have either a quick Botox or Restylane touchup, or go the full distance and book a tummy tuck or breast augmentation procedure, they do so with knowledge of the cosmetic surgery procedures of celebrities in mind. From media speculation over Robert Redford's alleged face-lift to Courtney Love's reported eyelift, from Victoria Beckham's breast enlargement to Sharon Osbourne's $700,000 splurge on surgical procedures, including DD breast implants, celebrity plastic surgery is endlessly debated in the media – discussed, dissected and desired. How much surgery celebrities have had, whether they need more, and the 'outing' of celebs that have not had surgery but should, all form part of the staple diet of current media and popular culture.

Because popular media culture commands us to enjoy celebrity plastic surgery, it is also the social arena from which many ordinary people do a good bit of thinking regarding their own lives and its future possibilities. Celebrity culture thus speaks directly on certain basic concerns to do with the body, ageing and desire – managing, as it does now, to dismantle dramatically the traditional notion that one looks older as one biologically ages. In this sense celebrities, as Richard Dyer argues, 'become models of consumption for everyone in a consumer society'.[12] If our media culture is mad with desire for celebrity plastic surgery, seized by an insatiable lust for documenting and assessing cosmetic enhancements to celebrity bodies, this is because ordinary people are subject to such hypnotic powers, which constitute changing public perceptions about the relationship of the body and society.

If celebrity plastic surgery is a dominant symbol of Western capitalism, it is because it runs all the way down in current social attitudes – such that the human body is now thought founded on nothing but its own infinite plasticity. To the question 'How can I re-invent myself?', contemporary Western culture has tended to reply: 'Celebrity!' Celebrity is part cultural and part divine, and to this extent a pure image of creativity. The self-affirmative cast of celebrity culture, however, is routinely brought low by the celebrated themselves. Celebrity as a culture is littered from end to end with addictions, pathologies, neuroses, even suicides. But this is not the only disabling factor to those in search of imitating the alleged creative culture of celebrity. For to claim that self-reinvention can be staged through the imitation of celebrity culture involves, as it happens, a kind of 'double displacement' of reality. For one thing, this displacement occurs partly because what is copied – the celebrity, the hero, the god – is mere image (no more and no less). It is also a displacement because the idealized image of celebrity – and particularly celebrity bodies – cannot sustain the projections invested by ordinary people without resulting in an aggressive emotional deadlock (of which more shortly). Either way, what helps to found celebrity culture is the desire to imitate or copy, and this is turn depends on knowing the world and especially its media representations.

If knowing the world suggests immersion in the mass media and popular culture, knowing oneself involves this equally, if not more so. For only if one knows how others go about the business of interrogating their inner lives through, say, psychotherapy or psychoanalysis, will one be in a position to contemplate the doing of this for oneself. Someone who watches daytime talk shows about relationship infidelities or transgressions of intimacy confronts and considers a whole range of tacit rules governing sexuality and gender power. Someone who reads self-help books encounters various protocols pertaining to the management of personal problems. Such self-management and self-stylization is what the late Michel Foucault called 'care of the self' – the complex tacit or informal kinds of knowledge that individuals deploy in devoting attention to their self-conduct.[13] In our own time of digital media and reality television, knowing both self and the world means, among other things, *knowledge of celebrity culture*. Today, arguably, individuals increasingly take celebrities as objects of knowledge for both the representation and the conduct of social life. From the confessions of celebrities regarding the cosmetic procedures they have undergone to the celebrity marketing of designer dentistry or the rejuvenating effects of skin cream, the values of celebrity culture seduce people to conform to what is treated as beautiful or desirable. Celebrity and aesthetic value go hand in hand. In this sense, too, celebrity is the power of authenticating ways of living, certificating styles of self-presentation, and thereby inscribing the individual self in broader structures of power.

Celebrity and the masses, or fame and fandom, are not then the opposites that many critics seem to think them. If celebrity broadens to, and functions as, a culture, this is because it penetrates to the inner sanctum of human identity. Personal subjectivity in the media age is more and more fashioned in the image of celebrity culture, and the most palpable representation of that culture is probably cosmetic surgery and its technologies of plasticity. Even so, how is this golden age of celebrity cosmetic surgery internalized – that is, taken up and lived – by its subjects? How, exactly, do people come to identify with celebrity culture and its prizing of surgically enhanced beauty? Media theorists Donald Horton and Richard Wohl offer some instructive leads on this process in their argument that media communications promote 'para-social interaction'.[14] If mass-media communications extend interaction beyond the model of face-to-face encounters, this is because the media cuts across time and space and inaugurates a world of mediated, non-reciprocal interaction. Mediated forms of communication, in effect, 'unhook' participants from the standard obligations of face-to-face dialogue. As one critic comments: 'Today we live in a world in which the capacity to experience is disconnected from the activity of encountering.'[15] Mediated, para-social interaction is thus framed on only the impression of reciprocity, the illusion of egalitarian communication.

Horton and Wohl analysed the mass media during the 1950s. A great deal has obviously changed since that time. The corporate diversification of media networks, the arrival of video and subsequently DVD recorders, digital technologies and the Internet: these are just some of the changes that comprise the great media revolution of our time. Many are developments promoting increased levels of media interaction, of heightened para-social interaction. Indeed, it may seem plausible to think that the basic thrust of the thesis of para-social interaction remains valid, even if the concept is now increasingly stretched to breaking point. Consider, for example, reality television programmes such as *Cosmetic Surgery Live* and *Plastic Surgery: Before and After*, which broadcast detailed and often gruesome coverage of cosmetic surgical procedures. The telescoping of body-part enhancement presented by these programmes provides audiences with detailed, practical knowledge of cosmetic surgical culture. Such mediated communication can, in turn, be brought to bear on processes of appropriation – that is, when viewers decide to undergo forms of cosmetic surgery witnessed on television.

The thesis of para-social interaction takes us some distance in grasping the ubiquity of cosmetic surgical culture in our age of global communication networks. But, still, we need to ask about the emotional dimensions of people's appropriation of cosmetic surgery as mediated through popular and celebrity culture. We need to enquire about the kinds of imagined freedom, as well as debilitating fear and anxiety, that celebrity culture breeds. From the viewpoint of ordinary people, or fans, celebrity is routinely experienced as a realm of unconstrained possibility. For the fan, the celebrity is the one who is true, free, transcendent. To worship celebrity in this way is to *project* part of the self onto the *idealized other*, and thus to experiment with a safe – indeed hermetically sealed – fantasy of life's possibilities. As sociologist John B. Thompson has contended, fandom involves wrapping up a significant part of an individual's self-identity in an identification with a distant other (the celebrity), and negotiating the necessary shifts between the world of fandom and the practical contexts of daily life. From this angle, the fan's symbolic equations may run something like this: Celebrity – Money – Power – Happiness – Love. On billboards and movie screens the world over, celebrities are seen as those living the good life, and thus worthy of identification, desire and imitation.

And yet, for the fan at least, the world of celebrity brings with it an awkward contradiction. Celebrity culture may promise independence, but in order for the fan to access this sublime experience (even if only 'at a distance') she finds herself dependent on the idealized image of the screen world. This kind of dependency can be severely debilitating, such that the dividing line between fandom and fame becomes blurred. Etymologically, the term 'fan' is related to 'fanatic', and this is one reason why contemporary celebrity implicates its subjects in forms of obsessive thinking, mania and aggression. From this angle, fandom can become a kind of addiction, in which the celebrity is just a stand-in for the projection of aggressive, deadly passions towards idealized images – rather as John Lennon's murderer Mark Chapman remarked that he felt compelled to eradicate the 'phoney peace-loving' multi-millionaire ex-Beatle.[16]

If the relation between fandom and celebrity has a built-in element of fanaticism, this is intensified in the surgical world of cosmetically enhanced celebrity bodies. At its worst, media and everyday cultural scrutinizing of the surgical habits of celebrities borders on the terroristic. Popular culture is saturated with references to the sagging skin, wrinkling eyelids and cellulite of ageing stars, as well as their desperate surgical attempts to turn back the clock. The paparazzi use telephoto lenses to unmask the artificial enhancements of the rich and famous, revealing the flaws of Hollywood skin. And panic-stricken at the failures of celebrity culture to deliver on its promise of absolute freedom, media pundits deconstruct the defects of celebrity plastic surgery – from Farrah Fawcett's melted face-lift to Jordan's 34FF bursting breast enlargements. Such an aggressive brand of media scrutiny has the taste of fear about it – a fear that is, ultimately, corrosive of meaning. Virginia L. Blum, in *Flesh Wounds*, refers to this cultural trend as part and parcel of our 'sadistic anatomising fascination', in which a kind of fetishized, pornographic knowledge is obtained through following the cosmetic secrets of celebrity bodies.[17] Such knowledge is described as sadistic since it tends to adopt fragmenting perspectives of the human body, aggressively penetrating to the flaws of celebrity bodies.

In order to gain a better grasp of such forms of psychological torment, it is instructive to consider the emotional investments that ordinary people, or fans, make in celebrity. In identifying with celebrity culture an individual unleashes a range of fantasies and desires. The fan, through a psychological process termed projective identification, transfers personal hopes and dreams onto the celebrity. In doing so, good aspects of the self are psychologically experienced as *contained* by the other, the celebrity. In psychoanalytic terms, this involves *splitting*: the putting of good or desired parts of the self into something outside, or other, in order to protect such imagined goodness from bad or destructive parts of the self. And what goes for the individual also has application for the wider society. When affluent society produces a buoyant celebrity culture, in which people invest their considerable emotional energies in dreams of fame and fortune, its belief in the transcendent powers of stars is unbounded. Nothing appears beyond the celebrity world of privilege and glamour.

Like Freudian desire, celebrity obsession can become quickly disenchanted with itself – especially in a body-scrutinizing culture where images of celebrities are routinely 'outed' as flawed. Finding the picture-perfect celebrity body flawed appears traumatizing for many, a kind of sublimity gone awry. The problem, from a Freudian angle, is that the mechanism of projection enters into a form of antagonism with itself. In short, the fan – having projected desired aspects of the self onto the idealized other in order to keep destructive aspects of the self in check – discovers with shock these same human failings within celebrity culture itself. Media discussion about how high-definition TV will reveal Cameron Diaz's acne, speculation over Britney Spears's post-pregnancy blown-out stomach and telescopic photos of Goldie Hawn's cellulite: the imagined absolute power of celebrity is brought low by human frailty, the self-undoing and self-dissolution of the modern-day god of celebrity. There is, then, a powerful contradiction at work here. What has been denied or disowned through idealization of the artificially enhanced celebrity body – namely the frailty of the human body itself – comes back from the outside (in, say, media scrutinizing of celebrity flaws) as a painful intrusion into the world of the fan. This is a kind of return of the repressed. If previously celebrity stood for a kind of symbolic cheating of death (in the figure of the eternal youthful star), now it is apprehended as a reminder of the limits of self-fashioning. The rich and famous may lead the world in the culture of nip and tuck, but even they are ultimately undermined by the deathly body. At this point, the fan comes face to face with the emotional turmoil that an absorption in the world of celebrity was meant to protect against. From this angle, celebrity is indeed morbid, masochistic, perverse and deadly.

Even so, there is a way round this psychological conundrum, and for contemporary popular culture one pathway for avoiding the hauntings of celebrity consists in immersing oneself in consideration of the aesthetic appeal of body parts. That is to say, popular culture increasingly trades the dependency and disappointment bred by celebrity for the all-round enjoyments of celebrity body parts. This is why, at a cultural level, people can agree that Angelina Jolie's exaggerated lips are the new plastic surgery 'gold standard', without being overly concerned or preoccupied about, say, her relationship with Brad Pitt or the amount of children the star has adopted. Celebrity, of course, still triggers the broad social levels of interest in surgical self-reinvention it always did, but now with a focus on the surgically enhanced body part itself and less the career of the celebrity. On this view, it is Jennifer Lopez's bottom that is scintillating to modern branding and culture – whatever one may think of her singing. And, in the end, this is less an erosion than a transformation of celebrity and the frenzy of fame.

It is not only adults who follow the cult of celebrity to the operating theatre. Teenagers do as well. The mania for the surgical enhancement of the body in the image of celebrity culture has spread to adolescents, particularly girls. Thanks to the twin forces of new technologies and lowering costs, what used to be the preserve of wealthy, ageing women has now become a routine form of medical self-fashioning available to the many. In the case of adolescents seeking cosmetic surgery, the idea of imitating particular celebrity enhancements, of copying certain Hollywood body parts, is increasingly prevalent. Yet, perhaps shrewdly, many of today's young see that the best use of surgical culture arises not from reproducing celebrity but appropriating it.

'It's the start of the university year and an increasing number of teenage girls are starting the new term with bigger breasts, smaller bottoms and straighter noses', reports one newspaper conducting a journalistic investigation into cosmetic surgery.[18] An emergent societal tendency to respond to the body-image anxieties of teenagers through recourse to cosmetic surgery is noted by the newspaper, based on interviews and surveys conducted in 2007. 'The trend', according to journalist Sushi Das, 'is for liposuction or breast surgery between high school and university.'[19] Whilst some of today's young are satisfied with their looks or are sceptical of our celebrity-led surgical culture, there are many more profoundly dissatisfied and distraught. And it is the latter on which entrepreneurial surgeons and the cosmetic industries feed, transforming a teenager's anxieties into compulsions and, ultimately, addictions.

Surgical enhancement of the body, of course, is something that until very recently took place after a woman (or man) had lived in their skin long enough – and had imbibed enough media messages and cultural significations –not only to *feel* dissatisfied but to want to *do* something about it. Yet while surgery and sentiment remain closely allied, a new rite of passage is emerging. As natural beauty in the contemporary era is increasingly replaced by artificial beauty, the world of celebrity, for which art and the aesthetic are at one, moves to centre stage in the cultural promptings governing surgical culture. And the latest wave of this cultural current are teenagers seeking the dismembering of their inherited looks and reconstruction of their bodies as an end in itself.

In our hyper-individualist society in which money, sex and youth are celebrated, adolescents are supposed to be consumer savvy. Yet media pundits and cultural commentators routinely register alarm the moment that today's young act upon and are seen to enjoy the demands placed on them. This is child psychologist Michael Carr-Gregg, quoted in the newspaper investigation into cosmetic surgery mentioned above, on current trends in the self-reinventions of teenagers: 'What I'm seeing is this absolute cult of celebrity . . . I've got girls who want to look like Britney Spears, Christina Aguilera, but what they want above all is their sculptural appearance.' In our remorselessly image-conscious culture, everyone is urged to worship celebrity. And it is, indeed, adolescents on whose shoulders such crazed idealism lands especially hard.

Those who, like Carr-Gregg, denounce the beauty aspirations of today's youth do not grant much problematic weight to the ideology of celebrity. They simply dismiss it, as trivial or trivializing. Yet this is a marvellously duplicitous tactic, one that rides roughshod over the extent to which the medical profession is itself held in thrall to the cult of celebrity. For in the investigative journalist report into cosmetic surgery in which Carr-Gregg's comments appear, the individuals who emerge as most caught up in the possibilities of self-reinvention and extreme makeover are not adolescents but surgeons, psychologists and health professionals. Consider, for instance, the following reflection from Australian cosmetic surgeon Darryl Hodgkinson on the difference between aggressive cosmetic surgery and the help such surgery can provide to especially distraught teenagers. The example he offers is nothing as life troubling as severe facial scarring or skin burns, but rather concerns the *derrière*. There are, he comments, 'psychological consequences of having a real physical deformity like a really big fat bottom'. Since when, exactly, has a large bottom been rendered a 'physical deformity'? On the one hand, such a comment is launched from an allegedly value-free, medical base in which the ideology of celebrity is thought unable to cast its neurotic grip on life. On the other hand, the comment reflects celebrity culture to the core, with the white-knuckled intensity of a worldview that jerks its knee at a clothes size larger than zero.

Throughout this chapter I have explored a range of cultural and political factors that shape the meshing of celebrity and cosmetic surgical culture. Celebrity, I have suggested, not only repositions us in relation to our identities as changeable and revisable, but it also introduces a wholesale shift away from a focus on personalities to celebrity *body parts* and their artificial enhancement. To see the body in the light of celebrity culture is to see it in terms of possible surgical alterations. Self-expression becomes thus an instrument of imitation in our era of celebrity worship. Celebrity imitation, the most liquid of emotional forms, refers, of course, only to very particular audiences and fan communities. Most people in contemporary culture do not fully adopt such ideologies pertaining to the connection between plastic surgery and imitation. Indeed, many people remain quite ironic about these aspects of celebrity culture, acknowledging its trivializing impacts on the public sphere or fragmenting tendencies to wider cultural perceptions of the human body. Even so, irony of itself does not lessen the grip of celebrity worship upon the wider society.

This is, in fact, one new way in which people living in contemporary times differ from previous generations – that is, in terms of continual interpreting or ongoing scrutinizing of artificial enhancements of the body. 'The significant presence of cosmetic surgery in celebrity culture', writes Margaret Gibson, 'has created a media-driven practice of reading the body for signs of cosmetic surgery.'[20] Increased attention to the smallest details of skin, or the slightest alteration to body shape, is central to the way we now belong to media culture. This is obviously true of full-blown plastic surgery, where we ask: Has she or hasn't she undergone the surgeon's knife? We say to ourselves: surely he's had a face-lift or some work done – he looks younger than in his last film, doesn't he? But it is also true of augmented faces and bodies reliant on scalpel-free procedures. As Natasha Singer observes,

> the increasing popularity among celebrities of less invasive procedures has turned the idea of cosmetic treatments into a kind of guessing game played with equal gusto by red-carpet commentators and couch potatoes at home . . . The celebrity body has become a public document available for close reading and open to group interpretation.[21]

Such 'close reading' of celebrity skin is now increasingly common. Gary Lask, a clinical professor of dermatology at UCLA and author of a paper titled 'Cosmetic Dermotology: The Hollywood Perspective', notes that the beauty interventions of celebrities render it 'fun to speculate' who has undergone different treatments and to what gain. In this sense, we witness the emergence of widespread second-order reflections on the 'artificial beauty' of our bodies.

Such second-order reflections of the self – our scrutinizing of how we 'read' bodies – remains, however, a fraught affair. Part of the difficulty, of course, is that the body is not reducible to unambiguous readings. The scrutiny of celebrity bodies is a matter of keeping in play possible meanings, of seeing identity as relatively open-ended, and thus disclosing how the celebrated and wealthy interact with commercial cultures in order to transform and reinvent their selves. Even so, the activity of 'reading' celebrity culture and its augmented bodies is obscure and emotionally complex. Part of the difficulty arises from the *imaging* presented by techno-media itself. Again, Gibson is instructive here:

74

It is not necessarily easy to detect signs of surgical inter-vention, particularly in the case of magazine and website images where corrections of facial or other bodily 'flaws' might have been made by computer-graphic alterations rather than the surgeon's knife. The computer-graphic might even correctively rework the surgical correction.[22]

On this view, it is the media itself that gets 'in between' the celebrity and her or his interpreter, casting its technological shadow over the surgical alteration or transformation of the flesh.

In another sense, however, it is perhaps inadequate to lay blame solely on the media for the distortion, blocking or rewriting of celebrity images and their body transforma-tions. For if we acknowledge that it is body parts rather than the personalities of celebrities that now matter espe-cially to this new way of reading culture, then a different picture emerges. This is a much more pluralist and open-ended account of the soaking up of celebrity within cosmetic surgical culture. Certainly, a sharper sense arises of the psychological processes at work in the picking out and selection of different features of mediated celebrity bodies. This involves, for example, recognition of the complex focus changing that individuals bring to their participation in media culture, as people sometimes zone in on a partic-ular celebrity body disposition, or sometimes refocus on the cosmetically altered body as a whole. Some attempt to read cosmetic restructurings of the body in directly surgical terms, focusing on face-lifts, scarring, breast augmentation or pectoral implants. Others aim for a longer-term fix, look-ing at temporal discontinuities within presentations of the flesh, skin or celebrity surface.

In all these ways, individuals now engage with media culture in the *reading* of cosmetic surgical enhancements of the body. And not only celebrity bodies already surgically altered are subject to such readings. We read, too, for bodies that might have been transfigured, or for future possibilities of surgical alteration. For example, in 2006 – after much media speculation – pop diva Madonna admitted she had been thinking about visiting a plastic surgeon in an attempt to reverse the biological clock. 'I think about it like everybody', Madonna told Britain's *Daily Mirror*, 'and I don't rule it out'.[23] Close attention had been paid to the star's body throughout the media in the aftermath of the release of her album *Confessions on a Dancefloor*, in which the 47-year-old Madonna displayed her athletic body in several videos, prompting some media commentators to note that many women half the superstar's age could only dream of attaining such a gorgeous look. A frenetic chronicling of Madonna's lifestyle ensued, with media monitoring of all aspects of her lifestyle – from her three-hour daily exercise regime to her high-fibre and low-fat vegetarian diet. But, still, speculation was rife that she might have undergone the surgeon's knife. Images were carefully screened, photos appraised and interviews scrutinized. This labour of cultural reading received little or no support from the superstar herself. 'I am not going to hold a press conference if I have plastic surgery', she commented. But this only added fuel to the media fire.

The debate about the everyday reading of celebrity and its plastic world of self-reinvention is as much about the economy as about culture. John Gray claims that 'the cult of celebrity has become one of the chief drivers of the economy'.[24] This is no doubt true of celebrity marketing and media hype surrounding designer clothes and mobile phones, but it is also increasingly so as regards particular economies of self-improvement and self-enhancement. As Gray develops the point:

In an economy driven by the need to manufacture demand, fame sells everything else. This is most palpably true when anyone can be famous. What is novel about the entertainment economy is that it holds out the prize of fame to everyone. In the past, luxury goods were sold to the masses by linking them with the lifestyles of the famous. Today, it is the belief that anyone can be famous that sustains mass consumption. Celebrity has been made into a sort of People's Lottery, whereby the majority of people are reconciled to the tedium of their daily lives.

Indeed, this is more or less the opinion of everyone nowadays according to Gray: 'economic growth is sustained by the popular belief that we can all be winners in the lottery of fame'. To see the urge to fame as bound up with adopting the lifestyles of the celebrated is to acknowledge the triumph of cosmetic surgical culture. But cosmetic surgical culture, like other such ideologies of instant self-transformation, not only scoops up the world of celebrity. It is also anchored in the whole new capitalist system, to which Gray rightly draws our attention. An adequate account of cosmetic surgical culture needs to take into consideration such crucial links between the new economy, consumption and consumption patterns, a topic to which we may now turn.

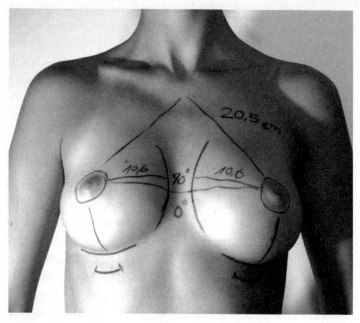

Preliminaries to a breast enlargement operation, 2007.

Chapter 3

Want-Now Consumerism: Immediate Transformation, Instant Obsolescence

The crunch came unexpectedly. Lauren had been catching up on episodes of *Desperate Housewives*, whilst thumbing through the latest edition of *Vogue*. As her attention wandered from the TV soap, her eyes fixed on a page that held her attention for the longest time. The alluring image of a young, attractive woman dominated the page. But it was the advertising hook that most seduced: 'The AUS$175 price tag is a lot less painful than an injection.' This was it: Lauren felt the pull of the long beckoning and alluring makeover she'd thought about for years. With *Desperate Housewives* rendered now just background noise, she read once again the product line: 'Botox-inspired Payot complex'. And the pitch. The ad read:

> The Dr NG Payot laboratories have drawn inspiration from cosmetics surgery and developed rides relaxes – a true dermo-relaxing, wrinkle-correcting skincare product. Based on neuro-cosmetics, this product boasts exceptional sensorial qualities. Its original combination of high-performance ingredients provides triple targeted action.

'What the hell,' thought Lauren, 'I'm going to do it.' Against her better judgement, she desired everything on offer – from 'botox-inspired' product to 'triple targeted action', from 'dermo-relaxing neuro-cosmetics' to 'wrinkle-correction skincare'. Oddly, it was this sales pitch for a beauty cream that was to become the defining moment. For Lauren, this was *her* tipping point. Her decision to undergo the surgeon's knife could not be otherwise explained. For like countless women of her generation, Lauren had leafed through the glossy magazines – *Elle*, *Marie-Claire*, *Cosmopolitan* – that advertised the promissory products of instant transformation. From the utopian claims for 'age rewind' to the comforting promise of 'cutaneous neuroprotection', Lauren felt part of a generation that accepted compounds, threads and potions as a means for the smoothing, tightening and remodelling of the body. Yet still there were other voices – seductive messages of interpersonal contact, evocative signals from the collective unconscious. That is to say, Lauren's decision to visit her cosmetic surgical centre should not be blamed on the media alone. Her decision rather reflects an ideology airborne: her impulse was part of a deeper cultural shift.

There are good reasons why Lauren should struggle to make sense of surgical culture at this point in her life. At 41 and having spent the better part of the last decade away from the workforce to raise her children, Lauren found herself pregnant once more. Whilst she and her husband, Tim, are far from prosperous, the couple had no hesitation in deciding to keep the existing family arrangements on course. Tim would continue as the principal bread-winner, whilst Lauren would stay at home with her children and new baby. After living their lives this way for many years, the option for Lauren to return to work wasn't really entertained. Money remains tight, but she describes things as manageable. In Lauren's case, at any rate, it is not so much cash as confidence that she craves. Above all, she wishes she could have her body back in shape; she wishes she could transform herself. As she puts it, 'I want to look good again, I want my self-esteem back.' Not that she regrets having had children.

And nor does she feel unloved or unwanted by her husband. But now, all these years later, thanks to several pregnancies and years of breast-feeding that have taken their toll, she feels the need to do something for herself. Something dramatic. 'To be honest', says Lauren 'I felt like I'd let myself go. How could Tim, or anyone, want me like this. In the end, I must confess, I knew I needed to resort to cosmetic surgery.'

Lauren, I learned, might have 'known' she would need to pay to get her body back, but her decision to undergo surgery was far from easy. She struggled, for many months after each pregnancy, with diets and exercise programmes. She toyed with the idea of cosmetic procedures and surgery, but instead would spend a 'fortune' on facials and creams. All the time, she felt pressure to 'improve'. Not from Tim, or her family. But rather society. 'Everywhere I looked', says Lauren,

> I saw 'yummy mummies' – taut and terrific. Then one day, after reading that ad I saw in *Vogue* (which was only for a face cream, but it got me so wound-up), I decided I was going to do it. To have the surgery.

The surgery that Lauren underwent transformed the 41-year-old's breasts from a B cup to a DD. This three-size jump transformed Lauren, she tells me, into a 'yummy mummy'. 'The surgery', she commented at our last meeting, 'has made me feel sensational. It's given me a real inner boost.' That boost came at the cost of almost AUS$15,000. And now that Lauren's confidence has returned, she's decided to take the process further.

> I came home from the hospital with an information booklet on related procedures, and on what I might consider to keep the 'new me' looking good. I'm already having Botox treatment every six months to hide my crow's feet. But now I think I'm going to have liposuction too. It's

taken only three months to decide this time, but I know I have the confidence to do this.

Some months after interviewing Lauren, I went to visit a day surgery that specialized in post-surgical check-ups for patients who had undergone cosmetic surgery. Talking with the patient relationship manager, Lisa, my understanding deepened of just how far down in our culture lies the obsession with cosmetic surgery. Before beginning my research for this book, I had assumed that surgical clinics and day centres would be mostly populated by the wealthy. As it happens, this assumption was quite wrong. Class differences, Lisa explained, were difficult to isolate. She saw patients from all walks of life. Some had plenty of money; others were prepared to borrow in order to transform themselves. It was also difficult to find factors such as age and relationship circumstances as definitive. Lisa saw many women in the age bracket of 18 to 30. But there were so many other categories of patients: older women, single mothers, women who had had children some years ago, divorcees. Cosmetic surgical culture at once seduces and cancels social differences.

Yet it seemed to me, reflecting on the work of this day surgery, that Lauren's story mimicked various social forces that are producing what I am calling cosmetic surgical culture. For one thing, the experience of her post-baby body was largely negative, shaped largely as it was by the cultural influences of family, media and popular culture. Lauren's fears about her post-baby body, and in particular feeling undesirable, relate in complex ways to the forms of consumption promoted by cosmetic surgery. It is just because cosmetic surgical culture has been so spectacularly successful in persuading so many women that breast implants, liposuction, tummy tucks and face-lifts are the road to a successful future that the fears and forebodings of people such as Lauren go all the way down – in both emotional and social terms. For another reason, Lauren's recasting of her life through the lens of cosmetic surgical culture reflects the increasing pressure on mothers to measure up to the new expectations of society, expectations arising from the social forces of cosmetic surgery, advanced technologies and the reinvention craze. The day-surgery patient manager, Lisa, told me that more and more women choose to have tummy tucks because they are unable to shift the excess skin generated through their pregnancy. Likewise, she noted that breast-feeding can lead to a loss of volume in the breast tissue, and one way to counter this is through breast implants. 'Because of the saggy skin', she comments acidly, 'some women need breast implants.' I'm struck by Lisa's use of the word 'need'. At the same time, this seems a reasonable description of the world and its options as they appeared to Lauren.

One way to understand the hopes, desires and frustrations of Lauren's experiments with cosmetic surgical culture is in the contradictions of consumerism. For the modern age, consumption emerges as the most sublime phenomenon, attempting to reconcile the apparently contradictory forces of desire and disappointment, beauty and terror. If there is something mesmerizing about consumerism it is not only because it trades in extravagant expectations, but because it also discards and deceives as well as seduces. At once promising scintillating satisfaction and yet frustrating fulfilment, consumerism inhabits a terrain of lethal ecstasy – each repeated frustration of desire helping to unleash, in turn, new wants and fresh appetites. A realm of deception, there is something always *excessive* about consumerism, and to that extent it represents both cultural continuity and anti-social rupture. In one sense, consumerism is enthralling, overwhelming, transgressive and traumatic. As such, it promises to lift one beyond the known world to a power of pure freedom and unconstrained selfhood. But in another sense, these fearful powers of the consumer society are brought low, rendered dazzlingly empty, by the frustration of fulfilment. Consumerism thus oscillates between the utopian immensity of its promises and the non-satisfaction rendered by its products.

Zygmunt Bauman writes of the current compulsive obsession with accumulating experiences and acquiring goods as an 'economics of deception'. Here is the sociological reasoning he gives in his book *Liquid Life:*

> Consumer society rests its case on the promise to satisfy human desires in a way no other society in the past could do or dream of doing. The promise of satisfaction remains seductive, however, only so long as the desire stays ungratified; more importantly, so long as there is a suspicion that the desire has not been truly and fully gratified. Setting the targets low, assuring easy access to goods that meet the target, as well as a belief in objective limits to 'genuine' and 'realistic' desires – that would sound the death knell of consumer society, consumer industry and consumer markets. It is the *non*-satisfaction of desires, and a firm and perpetual belief that each act to satisfy them leaves much to be desired and can be bettered, that are the fly-wheels of the consumer-targeted economy.[1]

The consumer's world is one of frustrated desires, dashed hopes; deceit – the broken promises of producers – is the *sine qua non* of consumerism and its ever-expanding terrain of new needs, wants and desires.

How does consumerism multiply itself? If deceit, excess and waste are built in to the functioning of consumer markets, what keeps people anchored in consumer culture? For Bauman, the consumer industry deploys two crucial strategies in keeping people orientated to its markets. The first consists in the *devaluation* of consumer products soon after, and increasingly as they near, saturation point in the market.

Yesterday's DVD player is today outperformed by digital recording; the mobile phone purchased recently from the high street is already out of date, supplanted by the new features of the latest stock. Such degradation of product durability, writes Bauman, goes hand in hand with the stimulation of new elements, designer markets and products. Moreover, this degradation of durability is nothing new; it is a method known to, and practised by, the consumer industry since its inception. What is new, however, is the dissolution in the time frame by which consumer products are thought to remain of lasting value. What used to last five years may be lucky now to last several months, such is the spread of transience throughout consumer culture. In the global intermeshing of human affairs, not least in as tumultuous a space as the service and technology sectors of the new economy, it is no easy matter to decide whether a purchased product is still relevant or desirable to today's lifestyle of accelerated consumption. For what the consuming self confronts is not simply some exterior set of guidelines regarding product or service durability, but those guidelines 'internalized' in the course of preparing oneself to be 'fully prepared' and 'always ready' for new consumer offerings, which now looms over individuals as a benchmark for measurements of the adequacy of the self. In today's society of consumers, the main task is

> to develop new desires made to the measure of new, previously unheard-of and unexpected allurements, to 'get in' more than before, not to allow the established needs to render new sensations redundant or to restrain the capacity to absorb and experience them.[2]

The second strategy developed by the consumer industry for the stimulation of consumer's desires, according to Bauman, is more subtle, yet effective. This consists, he explains, in 'the method of satisfying every need/desire/want in such a fashion that it cannot but give birth to new needs/desires/wants'.[3] This kind of exploiting of consumerist attitudes involves the continual cross-referencing of products, labels, brands and services. When people come to buy things, consumer marketing is now at work (and overtime) to ensure that the product on offer does not result in the *closure* of the consumer's consumption of goods. This it does through the *linking* of products and services with other consumer options. The consumer of skincare moisturizer, for example, may wish to re-energize their skin, but in shopping for the desired product they are likely to be cross-referred to endless related products – UV protection, pure ginseng extract creams, vitamin E and C products – all sold with the marketing hype of 'how to look radiant'. The capacity to keep all consumer options open, the willingness to embrace the fluidity and cross-currents of market-supplied services and substances: these are the crucial traits of contemporary consumption. 'Desire', writes Bauman, 'becomes its own purpose, and the sole uncontested and unquestionable purpose.' Such desire is that which feeds spontaneity in shopping – the desire not simply to consume more, but to consume the endless possibilities offered by the consumer industries for the reconstruction and reinvention of the self. As Bauman reflects: 'The code in which our "life policy" is scripted is derived from the pragmatics of shopping.'[4]

Still I wondered whether Lauren's observation about the link between the marketing of beauty products and the ideologies of cosmetic surgical culture held true for other women and men. I also wondered whether such advertising strategies matched Bauman's analysis of the consumer industry. Some time after Lauren and I last talked, I went back to the transcripts of her interviews. I was struck, re-reading these, with the very sharp lines she drew between the advertising of beauty products on the one hand and her decision to undergo the surgeon's knife on the other. Like almost all women of her age in cities of the West, Lauren felt a pressure to measure up to the norms promoted by the beauty industries. And, as it transpired, she felt this pressure intensely.

I decided to explore further the advertising campaigns for beauty products in order to understand Lauren's experience better. Leafing through various women's magazines at the local library, I found the following advertising pitches for beauty products:

> '*Surgery can wait! You laugh, you frown, your brow furrows . . . your skin contracts and wrinkles deepen. Our solution? Wrinkle De-Crease*'

> '*Pump it up 40%: Up to 40% Plumper Lips Collagen Effect*'

> '*Try the latest advances in non-surgical facelift treatment*'

> '*My Lips Are In Perfect Shape: My Lips Look Fabulously Full and Perfectly Contoured*'

> '*As good as surgery: airbrushed perfection in an instant*'.

The language is hypnotic in its explicit, or sometimes half-conscious, referencing of all things surgical. From the perspective of the consumer industry, women are beautiful to the extent that the *project* of anti-ageing and its marketed strategies are adopted and followed. Consumer society requires a salutary stiffening of the resolve of individuals: to knuckle down and reverse all signs of ageing, to identify and destroy indications of mortality. In consumer society, these strategies may be many and varied, but they increasingly draw inspiration from and reference cosmetic surgical culture.

Thinking sociologically about these advertisements, and about their promise to mitigate and reverse the daily torments of ageing for women in an ageist society, I felt I could understand better the things that had so preoccupied

Lauren. She had been, for example, troubled by the number of women in magazine ads who showed no sign of bagging under their eyes. 'I find I can get 50 or so pages in the thick monthly glossies', she told me, 'before seeing a woman with a line.' She was troubled by the need to find which skincare product was the right one for her to reverse the signs of age-ing successfully. She was, in fact, troubled by a whole host of things: her appearance, sexuality, blotchy skin, ageing cleav-age. Yet her troubled mind was unable to make the leap to think critically about skincare products geared to the anti-ageing market. If anything, she felt her capacity to think had itself been attacked, assaulted, brought low. Seduced by the promises of advertising, she found herself thinking within the frames of reference set by the marketing industry – with its heavy stress on the powers of cosmetic surgical culture.

This is not to say, of course, that it is all the 'fault' of con-sumer markets and the consumer industry. One reason why the marketing strategies for skincare products – with all the referencing to cosmetic surgical culture that I have noted – are so successful is that the promises on offer are what people *want* to hear. Indeed, it is what many people *crave* to hear. Consumer society thus both draws upon and represses the basic anxieties that our culture inaugurates in respect of youth, ageing and mortality. The anxiety that women like Lauren feel about their beauty and sexiness, in other words, somehow becomes inscribed within the soothing marketing promise that signs of ageing can be reversed. At once held in thrall to surgical culture and morally removed from it, the avid reader of women's magazines tracking the latest advances in skincare products is as much a fanatic in her own way as the consumer who subscribes to *Cosmetic Surgery Monthly*. And indeed, as Lauren was to discover, the line separating these realms is precariously thin.

Naomi Cambridge and her boyfriend, Steve, were reported in 2005 by London's *Evening Standard* as 'the vainest couple in Britain'.[5] The reason? The couple spend, on average, £20,000 a year on their looks and acknowledge they are 'cosmetic surgery addicts'. Naomi's flawless complexion, the article notes, has been maintained through adherence to a beauty regime that comprises three Botox sessions and four skin peels annually, the regular whitening of her teeth and the treatment Lipo-Melt (which involves the injection of a soya-based product into fatty areas of the body in order to reduce visible signs of fat). Perhaps more graphically than for many, cosmetic surgery encapsulates for Naomi the thrills and spills of life in a consumer-driven society. Acknowledging to the *Evening Standard* that cosmetic surgery is addictive, she comments:

> I don't want to look unnatural. I probably will have a face-lift when I'm much older. I just want to enhance what I've got and I don't see anything wrong with that. It's the same as changing your hair colour.

Everything about cosmetic surgical procedures seems to seduce and is exciting, yet, as she comments, people do not want to look 'unnatural'. Yet how one might tell the 'natural' from the 'unnatural', the 'beautiful' from the 'artificial', remains puzzling in this context.

The link between exciting experiments and foreboding fears that I mentioned may not yet be clear enough, although doubt and anxiety are certainly evident in Naomi's acknowledgement that she's only biding her time until a facelift. The psychologically attuned reader of the *Evening Standard* article on Naomi's consumption of surgical culture might, however, spot the deeper source of her fears and forebodings – which primarily revolve around her boyfriend, Steve. According to the article, Steve is quick to point out the dangers of particular foods (such as chocolate), worrying about cellulite. He also emerges as sharply critical of Naomi's appearance, encouraging the non-invasive procedures she undertakes to maintain her looks. As Naomi says of Steve: 'He's had a lot of very attractive girlfriends and can be quite critical of me.'

While hardly the most attractive portrait of her partner, it transpires that Steve's own cosmetic surgery regime is equally striking, if not more so. Among his annual beauty maintenance spending of £8,000, he undertakes Botox four times a year, Lipo-Melt six times a year, Hydrafill implants (the injection of gel into wrinkles that produces a smoothing result), as well as skin peels and other beauty treatments. The man, it seems, dwells within a kind of permanent bodily reconstruction unit, one in which more and more cosmetic consumer purchases are accumulated.

Although the *Evening Standard* article about Naomi and Steve is far from the extreme end of 'extreme reinvention', there is something pathological about the obsessive search for bodily maintenance and reconstruction that it reports. What is pathological is not the desire for body-part enhancements, since cosmetic surgical culture, as I have sought to demonstrate, is increasingly rendered a 'necessity' (and is thus normalized) in contemporary societies. Rather, the suggestion that we are dealing with pathological symptoms is premised on my argument that cosmetic surgical culture provokes the very anxiety it seeks to quell. Security for the body means fending off every sign of ageing or maturity, and such defensive measures are principally undertaken through consuming surgical culture. Yet cosmetic surgical enhancements, as Naomi and Steve know only too well, are not designed to last. Cosmetic surgical products have a very short shelf life, which is one reason why people quickly feel dissatisfied with the procedures they have. What makes cosmetic surgical culture addictive is that it is this very failing that incites people to buy more products and procedures. This is why fantasy is so pivotal to surgical culture, from the advertiser's pitch of 'the perfect body' to the constructing of beauty in the eye of the cosmetics vendor.

Cosmetic surgical culture thus brings intense disappointment as well as excitement and hope in its wake. Potent fantasies that revolve on a smoothed, tightened and remodelled body deflate at the same time as they inflate people's emotional lives. The body becomes magically transformed through various 'non-invasive' procedures that inject liquids, compounds and threads, while the individual's sense of identity, framed on a reflexive awareness that such 'enhancements' will turn to waste, splinters on the repeated frustration of desire. Still, the intoxicated fantasies of potency and possibility in which the consumer industry trades are the things that most galvanize the passions of consumers. In our fast-flowing, mobile, even liquid world, cosmetic surgical culture promotes a fantasy of the body's infinite plasticity. The message from the makeover industry is that there's nothing to stop you reinventing yourself however you choose. Yet your surgically enhanced body is unlikely to make you happy for long. Surgical enhancements of the body are primarily undertaken with the short term in mind. They are 'until the next procedure'.

Caught in a brutally despairing circle, the individual's consumption of cosmetic surgical culture appears incapable of coming to an end. A further reason for this urge to makeover is that the desire to remake selfhood becomes semi-autonomous, the very act of surgical enhancement of body parts becoming an object of desire in itself. It is this deadly repetition that means 'surgery addicts' are unable ever to know how much surgery is enough. In any event, this is not a problem for consumer marketing and the consumer industry. The more uncertainty and anxiety the beauty industry creates, the more hungry individuals become for 'expert' solutions to cosmetic dilemmas. Accordingly, when people acknowledge that they 'need' cosmetic surgery – no doubt after many soul-searching hours of looking in the mirror – they routinely do so through succumbing to the advice of cosmetic experts, with their battery of procedures and products.

Here is where consumerism enters the picture. Consumer society and the consumer industry fit perfectly into cosmetic surgical culture, as the new economy is so well attuned to selling products, procedures and services to the anti-ageing market. From the advertising of skincare products to cosmetic surgery magazines, the message of popular culture is that personal makeover is progressive, even beneficial. The consumption of cosmetic surgical culture is the celebration of personal change. Crucially, people crave to hear such messages. That is to say, there has been an attentive and widespread public response to the new economy – so much so that it seems there is something normative about the kind of transgression promoted by cosmetic surgery. Surgical enhancements of the body may be surplus to our biological needs, but it is this very supplementary excess that makes cosmetic surgical culture intoxicating.

If there is consumer culture at work here, there is also consumer identity – as we have seen with Naomi and Steve, who energetically devote themselves to the bodily reconstruction of the self. The kind of identity bred by cosmetic surgical culture, however, is far from nourishing or self-sustaining. This, to be sure, is partly the result of the eradication of the long term – the eclipse of the 'forever' – in cosmetic surgical culture. Botox may make you look younger, but it is hardly likely to foster an appreciation of human frailty or finitude. The whole commercial language of cosmetic surgical culture is relentlessly focused on episodic change, the purchase of one-off transactions. Cosmetic procedures – from Botox and collagen fillers to liposuction and breast augmentation – are increasingly reduced to a purchase mentality. There's now an emergent generation of consumers who might be called the Plastic Generation, who treat cosmetic surgery as on a par with shopping: consumed fast and with immediate results.

Even so, the question remains of how society goes about *preparing* consumers – cajoling, seducing and enticing them – for the culture of cosmetic surgery. Ideas about the exploitation of consumerist attitudes may take us so far, but still I wonder if such accounts don't simply reduce the individual to a passive cipher of cosmetic surgical culture. As in Marx's theory of ideology, the individual in many recent accounts of consumerism appears as little more than the plaything of wider social forces.[6] Advertising is quite often demonized in this connection, as a corrosive force that promotes self-fashioning without self-understanding. However, such a viewpoint doesn't tally with the individuals I've encountered and spoken with regarding cosmetic surgical culture. It doesn't adequately engage with their experiences of cosmetic surgery, neither the benefits nor damages. In the broadest sense, cosmetic surgical culture promotes forms of identity experienced both as creative and destructive, life affirming and death dealing. As such, the consumer of cosmetic surgical culture emerges both as victor and failure, winner and loser.

Consumer culture may drive an individual to see the surgical enhancement of the body as a desirable goal or positive outcome; yet in doing so the consumer will need to make all sorts of complicated reckonings, based on reflexive assessments of competing products and procedures, about cosmetic surgery. None of this is necessarily straightforward, and the decision to undergo a surgical procedure or service cannot be taken for granted. Whilst the advertising of cosmetic surgery and makeover culture overreaches itself, the choosing of products and procedures is always a much more pragmatic affair. Think of, say, Lauren's long drawn-out engagement with the beauty consumer industry, her agonizing over what was right for her. Certainly, advertising and marketing played a vital role here, but there was nothing inevitable about her decision to undergo the surgeon's knife.

The foregoing reflections about consumer ambivalence touch on a contradiction that goes to the very heart of the consumer industries, and thus is noteworthy for the analysis of cosmetic surgical culture. Consumption, in both its personal and social dimensions, is founded on the West's obsession with freedom – which is often and increasingly taken to mean *freedom of choice*. An individualist society requires an especially well-entrenched ideology that the consumer can make her life however she chooses, transforming identity in the very act of such decision-making. In the case of material consumption, this ideology regularly takes the form of the so-called rational expression of wants. In principle, the market sets limits to the expression of 'realistic' wants. In reality, such wants are shot through with consumerist hopes, dreams and desires. Consumerism is overshot, as it were, by consuming passions. Most of us know that desire cuts deeply into economic life, but many (largely economists and policy makers) choose to ignore the ramifications of this. Instead, the rationalist thesis asserts the primacy of rational choice and the free-market arts of self-choosing: the reflexive consumer, we are told, makes a calculated assessment, after careful scrutiny of competing products, and the shopper is in turn rewarded for her diligence through the acquisition of the much sought-after consumer object – a new dress, car or holiday. But such consumer satisfaction, of course, lasts only briefly, perhaps just for a moment. To be sure, there is strenuous shopping and flights of fancy, there is the pleasure of unregulated gratification, even enchantment, but it is rarely freedom to rise above the ideology of the market itself. Consumerism is thus often at odds with genuine autonomy, with the creative reckoning of one's own capacities. Maybe this is why consumerism breeds intense restlessness.

In this sense, to speak of the consumer's freedom of choice is a kind of performative contradiction, since multinational capitalism and the new economy are so adept at fashioning needs, desires and appetites that people never knew they had. Consider, once again, skincare beauty products. From stressed-out skin to dull hair, marketers of skincare products play relentlessly on women's (and often men's) insecurity about their looks. Imaging skin defects, and particularly magnifying their potentially disastrous social consequences, is vital to the selling of beauty products – many of which are, in any event, ineffective or of doubtful value. According to the BBC's *The Money Programme*, for example, the average British women will spend approximately £183,000 on beauty products during her lifetime. The irony of such large expenditure is that few of the women surveyed by the BBC believed that these skincare products did very much. Interestingly, most of the products reviewed were at the more 'extreme' end of beauty products – from claims to 'redensify skin' to 'collagen effect' gloss. But we need to remain attentive to what factors induced these women to spend large sums of money on beauty products. Some women admitted that they bought very expensive beauty products simply because they were costly, and thus exclusive. Many other women acknowledged that they had purchased a product because an advertisement or beauty expert had made reference to it in the selling of another product.

Such market cross-referencing of products and services within the beauty industry finds an interesting parallel in cosmetic surgical culture, where the consumer is presented with many different options and possibilities as a means of complementing and legitimating experiences of cosmetic surgery already consumed. Any patient or client returning from a cosmetic procedure performed by a top surgeon in, say, Harley Street or Beverly Hills is today likely to do so with more than mere bandages and wounds. Increasingly, cosmetic surgeons dispatch their patients home with a brochure, catalogue or DVD – in which is outlined other cosmetic procedures by which one can keep one's surgically enhanced body up to scratch. In marketing terms, this involves deflecting attention from the particular procedure undergone and broadening the advertising coverage to encompass the barrage of procedures now offered by cosmetic surgical culture. In this way, the market for cosmetic surgery is maintained through selling its associations, linkages and possibilities.

One recent advertisement for cosmetic surgery in Australia, for instance, presented multiple options for the consumer (from breast lifts and implants to liposculpture to facial rejuvenation), adding financial inducements for the purchase of procedures. The boxed, cut-out coupon advertising read thus: 'Bring in this voucher and save $$: Buy 1 body area and get one free.' Of course, in business terms this is clever marketing. But from the standpoint of the individual and wider society, such advertising may pose acute challenges and risks. It is not only the sheer number of procedures and services that stimulate and entice consumers here that may be of concern, or the broader medical or health-related issue of whether it is appropriate to encourage individuals to undertake multiple cosmetic and surgical procedures simultaneously. What is of more pressing sociological concern is the deflection of attention away from the actual *object* of cosmetic surgery: namely, the individual self. Put more specifically, the consumer, released from any deeper worry about the self, is free to choose new procedures for different 'body areas'. In this imaginary construct, the experience of cosmetic surgical culture is 'scrambled', through a process in which the consumer can change constantly the 'frame' of possibility whilst disengaged from wider personal and social considerations. After all, this is the whole point of cosmetic surgical culture: it encourages you to fantasize and desire cosmetically enhanced 'body areas'.

To be inside and outside the frame of the advertising illusion – to fantasize a position while remaining still on the margins – is central to the selling of extreme reinvention. And I have been struck, time and again, at the resourcefulness of many surgical clinics and cosmetic day centres in this connection. Some seek to entice the individual to enter the experience of cosmetic surgery with basic bribes: 'Free Consultation with Surgeon'. Others attempt to rope in potential clients by underscoring multiple possibilities. Such ads tend to focus on 'before and after' photos, with little in the way of text, thereby changing the consumers' positioning, from procedure to procedure. Again, 'bonus offer' advertising illustrates this. Such marketing is well reflected in the following advertisement – randomly selected from a *Health and Body* newspaper supplement:

> book and pay a deposit for liposuction / liposculpture in May and receive a fixed price of $12 per unit for Anti-Wrinkle injections for one whole year!

The selling of extreme reinvention and its associations – buy liposuction and get Botox free – seek to limit in the consumer's mind any linkage between cosmetic surgery and personal identity. For a body-obsessed and body-centred culture, the selling of cosmetic surgery involves no more and no less than trade in new procedures, novel experiences, new body parts.

Yet this deflection from self to body, a crucial trend in contemporary advertising all the way from clothes to cars, has its limits too. Trying out new strategies to make your body more youthful, fitter or sexy in appearance is not always as hassle-free as it seems. For much of how we now think about and experience the human body is embedded in deeper cultural anxieties over mortality, finitude and death. As Chris Schilling, a noted sociologist of the body, explains:

> We now have the means to exert an unprecedented degree of control over bodies, yet we are also living in an age which has thrown into radical doubt our knowledge of what bodies are and how we should control them.[7]

The 'radical doubt ' of which Schilling speaks is some-times enlivening, shifting personal life in a more experi-mental direction; but it is also proving most damaging, at least as far as issues to do with emotional literacy and the self-understanding of individuals are concerned. In a culture in which every aspect of identity can be instantly transformed, or the body endlessly remoulded, what is it that now grounds human decision-making about what is worth doing and why? There is now a technological vortex at the heart of current social, cultural and medical debates about the body, of which cosmetic surgical culture is a prime instance.

Reflecting on Lauren's encounter with surgical culture brings home just how emotionally crippling this intimate link between technology and the body can be. The com-mercially driven quality of Lauren's initial consumption of cosmetic surgery has already been noted. She looked to cosmetic surgery, prodded by beauty product advertising with strong surgical inflections, to resolve matters of personal insecurity about her appearance and looks. Given her satisfaction with the results of the breast augmentation, at first I thought that would probably be the end of Lauren's surgical spree. Yet, like countless others, she experienced a powerful conflict between remaking her body and the possibilities for further remoulding. Grasping this conflict, I realized that for Lauren there could be no return to traditional ideas of ageing gracefully; the world that once instructed women to accept the passing of time had now unravelled before her eyes, and she was not going to be left behind.

But if women like Lauren need freedom and the future, they also need guidance and instruction on how to make the most of their lives. This is perhaps why Lauren set so much store by the information booklet she brought home from the surgery. Now that she is well versed in which other surgical options might suit her lifestyle ambitions, she is – she tells me – more confident about her future. But there is nothing easy about her decisions concerning future cosmetic surgery. For the technological cult of surgical culture makes the remoulding of 'body areas' highly specialized and complex in this respect. At this Lauren drifts from a concern with self to body, from the personal to the impersonal. The problem itself is emotionally crippling.

Sharyn Hughes, 32, a successful hairdresser with several up-market salons across London, lay on a couch reading a holiday brochure. Her partner, Grant, a 27-year-old lawyer, had urged her to book an exotic holiday. Both Sharyn and Grant were hard-working and very highly motivated. It was always difficult to find time to go away, and even more difficult to synchronize 'relationship time'. But for this year, the couple had decided really to splurge – on a tropical holiday to Malaysia.

Not that Sharyn and Grant were unused to spending big on themselves. Expensive holidays, sports cars, designer clothes: these and other expensive items were all regular purchases in the Hughes household. Yet the Malaysian exotic holiday was radically different from anything the couple had done before. For in addition to five-star hotels, fine dining and exotic beaches, Sharyn would also undergo the surgeon's knife for a breast enlargement procedure, liposuction and designer dentistry, and Grant too would have liposuction and some cosmetic dentistry. Sharyn contemplated the advertising brochure from Makeover Getaways:

> Our Malaysian Makeover Package is a brilliant combination of surgery treatments, sunny beaches and shopping. Offering the latest technological facilities in an exceptionally clean hospital environment, and with guaranteed five star hotel accommodation for postoperative recovery and holiday, you will return home fully revitalized and looking wonderful.

From an economic point of view, the trip was enticing. The surgeries, accommodation, transfers and tour of Malaysia, all arranged by Makeover Getaways, would cost Sharyn and Grant a total of £9,000. The price also included medical consultations, surgeries, medication and associated hospital fees. For Sharyn and Grant, this represented exceptional value – since the cost of the medical treatment alone in the UK would have been in excess of £11,000.

Sharyn was no stranger to cosmetic surgical culture. In London, she had tried Botox – and, indeed, it now formed part of her routine personal makeover every four months. But the trip to Malaysia represented a more profound experiment: it linked her long-standing desire for a breast enlargement with her perceived need to 'get rid' of certain problem areas through liposuction. 'I figured', Sharyn commented, 'that I needed a thorough overhaul. And if I was going to do it, and go through all the associated pain, then I might as well get the five-star recovery in an exotic location.'

Sharyn and Grant returned to London from their surgical package trip feeling fabulous; 'we look great, and feel much younger!', she beamed. As it happens, the couple's experiment with sun, sand and surgery reflects part of much broader social changes occurring throughout surgical tourism today. The number of surgical tourists in Malaysia has more than doubled in recent years, rising from approximately 40,000 people in 2003 to more than 100,000 in 2006. Asia in general remains the world's hotspot for surgical tourism, particularly Thailand, Singapore and India.[8] Growing excellence in the performance of Western cosmetic surgical procedures, along with the growing globalization of staff within the corporate hospital chains across Asia, has driven the expansion of international patients. Bangkok's Bumrungrad International Hospital, for example, advertises that all its staff speak English, that it has hired more than 200 surgeons certified in the United States, and that it employs in excess of 70 interpreters. Similarly, Thailand's Phuket Hospital offers the service of interpreters in more than fifteen languages, and currently has an international patient base of approximately 20,000 people a year. But it is not just Asia that has thrived. Eastern European countries (such as Hungary, Latvia and Lithuania), Latin America, the Caribbean states and parts of the Middle East – notably Dubai, but also Bahrain and Lebanon – have all witnessed a dramatic rise of surgical tourism. As one commentator notes:

> Dubai has just built Healthcare City (DHCC) to capture the Middle East market and try and divert it from Asia. Unable to compete on price the Middle East has largely competed on quality, with Dubai bringing in German doctors to guarantee high skill standards, and Lebanon stressing its many doctors trained in Europe and America.[9]

Medical tourism took off dramatically during the late 1970s, due to the conjoined forces of low foreign currencies and cheap medical care. The rapid growth of medical tourism as a niche industry, writes John Connell, has arisen from

> the high costs of treatment in rich world countries, long waiting lists (for what is not always seen institutionally as priority surgery), the relative affordability of international air travel and favourable economic exchange rates, and the ageing of the often affluent post-war baby-boom generation.[10]

These trends have been dubbed 'the unlikely child of new global realities',[11] and have become more recently part of more complex patterns of global travel and consumption. What we see occurring today are the emergence and consolidation of territorial concentrations of cosmetic and surgical specialities, as countries around the world compete to provide medical and technological infrastructure that affords wealthy Westerners opportunities to undergo cosmetic surgery away from the routines of daily life at home. In providing medical infrastructure, as well as ensuring a steady supply of anaesthesiologists, medications, post-operative care facilities and so on, companies specializing in cosmetic package trips are creating new patterns of medical tourism and cosmetic standards of global surgery. In effect, this involves a 'lifting out' of cosmetic surgical culture from its embeddedness and visibility in the global cities of the West – London, Paris, New York, Tokyo, Sydney – and relocation to other low-wage spots around the globe. From this angle, new patterns of global travel and consumption opened up by surgical tourism are bringing together some of the most and the least privileged people across countries. Privilege in this context increasingly hinges on mobility. As surgical package holidays become larger in operation, more global, so the immobilities of local communities and workers on the ground of the destination country become more pronounced. Saskia Sassen has noted that the increased geographical dispersal and mobility of today's affluent goes hand in hand with 'pronounced territorial concentrations of resources necessary for the management and servicing of that dispersal and mobility'.[12] Similarly John Urry, a sociological pioneer in the study of mobilities, argues:

> What is significant is that as people and artefacts become more mobile, other people and objects become relatively less mobile. Overall the greater the extent, range and significance of mobility around the world, the more elaborate and complex the consequential patterns of immobilisation.[13]

These insights apply well to thinking about the large-scale immobile infrastructure supporting Sharyn's and Grant's surgical holiday in Malaysia. From flight attendants to hospital cleaners, from hotel staff to nurses, there are very large numbers of workers involved in assisting, checking, monitoring, providing hospitality, customer service, ground transportation and so on. Such workers, and the economic and social processes in which they are implicated, are not incidental to the phenomenon of surgical holidays; they in part help to constitute it.

To be sure, tourist travel is now the largest industry in the world, accounting for 11.7 per cent of world GDP, 8 per cent of employment and 8 per cent of world export earnings.[14] Such tourist mobilities are truly global in scope. It is estimated, for example, that there are more than 700 million international journeys made throughout the world each year, a figure that some analysts estimate will rise to more than one billion in the near future.[15] Such rising social and geographical fluidity – the increasing ability of people to travel long distances – is also a crucial factor in the globalization of cosmetic surgical culture. The advent of surgical safaris and cosmetic package trips is not only reorienting and transforming medical institutions throughout various sectors of the globe, it is restructuring old patterns of labour – from unskilled young workers to care providers and nurses. The associated realm of work stemming from medical tourism – involving ground-transfer providers, hotel cleaners, hospital attendants and so forth – arises from this growing globalization of cosmetic surgical culture. In *Tourism Mobilities*, Mimi Sheller and John Urry argue that

> there is an incredible range of employment now found within global tourism. Most people across the globe cannot fail to be implicated within, or affected by, these circuits of tourism and travel. Such employment includes travel agencies; transportation; hospitality; bars, clubs and restaurants and cafés; architecture, design and consultancy; media to circulate images through print, TV, news, and the internet; arts and

sports events and festivals; and NGO campaigns for and against tourist developments. The growth of the tourism industry also more widely reshapes patterns of urbanization, or infrastructure development (roads, airports, ports), or agriculture and food importation, of cultural production and performance, with implications for almost every economic sector.[16]

Recovering from her breast enlargement procedure at a private clinic in Malaysia, Sharyn might well have reflected on how she could have still been in the UK. Or the United States, or Australia. Or, for that matter, in any plush hospital throughout the polished West. For the exceptionally clean and sterile facilities in which Sharyn experienced her post-operative care had been designed to mirror, if not surpass, the standard of private hospitals and medical clinics around the world. Such design and management of the post-operative care environment helps to universalize private hospitals, but it also transforms such institutions into what Marc Auge has termed 'non-places': placeless, indistinguishable, indistinct.[17] Like shopping malls and airports, private medical facilities and clinics are increasingly indistinguishable; they are, in effect, designed as 'recuperative comfort zones' and organized around various kinds of medical and technological processes. One dominant aspect of the contemporary world is the so-called globalization of place, of locales and the built environment, and this is arguably true with the growing use of private clinics and medical institutions for the selling of surgical package trips. Well-run companies, specializing in medical and surgical tourism, provide a sense of 'global privatized enclosure' for the personal trials and tribulations of cosmetic surgery. Set within a medicalized environment, the patient recovering from cosmetic surgery in a private clinic rarely interacts in any sustained way with other patients or staff; at one remove from ordinary daily life, the hospital or clinic emphasizes a separate space or aesthetic in order for the patient to 'find their way back' to a more grounded or routine sense of self. The forces of globalization and high technology, available in the form of overseas private clinics and medical facilities, are producing 'entirely new experiences and ordeals of solitude, directly linked with the appearance and proliferation of non-places'. Understood in these terms, it is easier to see that Sharyn's luxurious solitude of post-operative care in a Malaysian private clinic was, in fact, a commercially purchased, private ordeal dominated by pain, bruising, antibiotics, sutures and scabby wounds. We know this is not the way surgical package trips are represented by the organizations themselves (and for obvious reasons), nor is it how patients often come to think about their overseas post-operative care. But, as I discovered in talking and listening to Sharyn and Grant, the cutting-edge technology and privileged medical conditions of surgical tourism could not hide the fact that much of their time overseas had been characterized by a kind of *solitary ordeal*. In the end, surgical tourism had deposited Sharyn on the other side of the world, without friends or family (and even without Grant, since he too was under the surgeon's knife), struggling to cope with, and recover from, invasive surgical procedures and their attendant unnecessary medical risks.

It's sometimes said that today's rapid globalization of medical tourism represents a dominant pathway for the future. In this scenario, the global elite jet off to exotic destinations, enjoying a combination of surgical rejuvenation and luxurious relaxation, only to return to their privileged lives looking ever younger, healthier and fitter. Despite the emphasis I have put on the transformative global developments associated with medical and surgical tourism, in my view such a scenario is unlikely to become the norm. For one thing, many people are rightly concerned about the risks and complications associated with medical procedures performed in foreign countries. The death of the

Nigerian First Lady, Stella Obasanjo, after undergoing liposuction and a tummy tuck in a private Spanish clinic on the Costa del Sol, is one recent high-profile case dramatizing the very high risks involved. Another factor tilting against the further spread of such developments concerns medical insurance. In general terms, neither personal nor travel insurance usually covers medical and surgical procedures carried out in foreign countries. That said, however, there are important ways in which the globalization of surgical package trips is creating new geographies of power between and within countries.

One way in which such changes are occurring lies in the consumer's conviction that not only is instantaneous gratification possible, but that neither time nor space significantly constrain the redesign or surgical enhancement of the body. Such a conviction is part and parcel of the inauguration by globalization of 'instantaneous time', the phenomenon of 'we want the future now'. Consumers today have the technological means of booking surgical holidays online, selecting discount international flights, going on shopping safaris – and all that such trips offer in the way of an imagined freedom instantly to reinvent the self. This involves, at the level of the individual self, an imagined temporal and spatial compression of the globe; the two-week surgical holiday to the other side of the world can be booked at a moment's notice, and undertaken in five-star comfort. Even if such fantasies neglect the realities, risks and pain of surgical holidays, as we have seen, they nonetheless serve to promote more fluid social identities.

A second, and related, way in which such processes are altering the fabric of contemporary social life lies in the reconfigurations of space, and particularly of the individual's withdrawal from everyday life into other, distant regions of 'recuperative space'. The single most important element in the consumption of surgical holidays lies in the consumer adopting a new attitude to social space – as a 'time out' from the ordinary, routine spaces of social life. Geographer Doreen Massey makes the case for taking space seriously in these terms:

> The fact that processes take place over space, the facts of distances, of closeness, of geographical variation between areas, of the individual character and meaning of specific places and repair – all these are essential to the operation of social processes themselves.[18]

Surgical holidays combine the consumer's originating country and the destination in a novel blend, involving imaginative and physical movement, proximity and distance, and new patterns of power and inequality as a result of the spatial restructurings of cosmetic surgical culture. Such unique layerings of social space, of proximity and distance, exert a profound emotional and personal sense of being 'outside time and space', or at least of being temporarily suspended from the daily rhythms of social life. These layers combine, I am suggesting, to create a privatized model of 'recuperative time and space' – in which the patient uses the destination country as a springboard to reconfigure mind and body before returning to the routine social spaces of home. As one commentator notes:

> For many what makes medical tourism so appealing is that no one need know there was anything medical about the trip. [One such couple from the US] visited South Africa a year ago for tummy tucks, liposuction and eyelifts. Back from South Africa they threw a Super-Bowl party. 'Friends kept saying we looked fantastic'. Funny how a good vacation can be such an uplifting experience.[19]

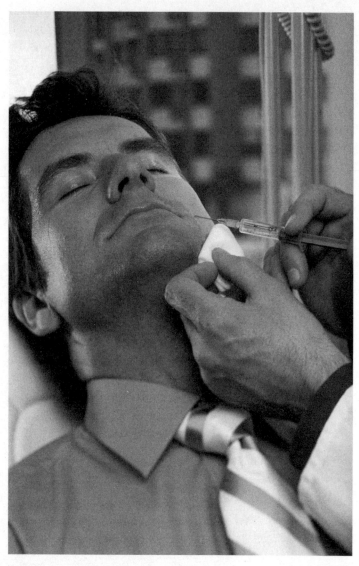

Man having a Botox injection, 2005.

Chapter 4

Making the Cut: Cosmetic Surgical Culture in the Global Electronic Economy

Richard Daley, as I will call him, is an American who came to London to work in the M&A division of one of the UK's leading investment banks. Since finishing his studies in Business Administration and Finance at an Ivy League college in the US, his career trajectory has been rapid. After a short period of training in the US, he worked for investment banks in Switzerland, Hong Kong and Australia. He welcomed the challenges of advising companies on capital markets and acquisition financing. He enjoyed the teamwork and fast-changing projects that arose from cross-border mergers and acquisitions. 'When you work in banking at such an advanced level, you will understand, the demands are very pressing and you develop intense relations with colleagues quickly – even though you're aware such projects are only transitory.' Now, in London, the short-term trajectory of deal making and teamwork is more evident than ever to Richard. He described to me the 'buzz' of the 24/7 investment-banking lifestyle – the thrills and spills of high-pressured work, the organizational challenges of no set daily routine.

For a man so seemingly at ease with the fluid world of global finance, I found myself surprised when Richard Daley told me how much he relished the firmly grounded nature of his morning routine at home, before leaving for the office. As it happens, he is anything but flexible when it comes to his domestic routine. Waking to BBC news on his digital radio at 6 a.m., the first thing Richard does each morning is to check his Blackberry for overnight email. I am most struck by the fixity of the ensuing ritual: he showers for fifteen minutes, from 6.10 to 6.25, and then dresses for the day. His clothing, from his selection of suits down to shirt, matching tie, cufflinks, socks and shoes, has all been chosen days in advance. Sitting in his minimalist kitchen by 6.45, drinking coffee and eating cereal, he scans the *Financial Times* to keep abreast of global finance. The routine, he tells me, doesn't vary – unless he is travelling. Such fixation on a set routine is partly what Freud meant by the notion of repetition compulsion, the endless replay of certain actions in order to keep complexity and ambiguity at bay and thus the assertion of some degree of control (however minimal) over the self and world.

Oddly, Richard hasn't followed this routine in recent weeks. Taking some time off from work, he told colleagues that he needed to get away for a break. Perhaps Paris. Maybe Vienna. The reality, though, is very different. Richard, 43, has been consulting doctors in Harley Street regarding cosmetic surgery. He decided he needed stomach lipo-suction. Rather than expressing any sign of guilt or anxiety over appearing vain, Richard speaks matter-of-factly, carefully explaining to me his reasons for undergoing the surgeon's knife. 'It pays to look good, everyone knows that', he remarks. And look good he always has, at least until quite recently. 'I've been reasonably fit all my life, but since I turned 40 I started to really balloon, developing a pot belly.' Richard tried to reverse his mid-life belly. Diets didn't work. Nor did trips to the gym. So it seemed quite natural to turn to cosmetic surgery, he tells me.

It seems, of course, absurd to think of cosmetic surgery as 'natural'. But there is a kind of logic to Richard's reason-ing here. If cosmetic surgery has come to represent a natural way of coping with the pressures of corporate life, this is above all because it has become a kind of 'manufactured nature'. Or, at least, this is what Richard seems to have in mind. Richard knows other investment bankers who have already had cosmetic work done, from Botox to chemical peels to mini-face-lifts. Noting how I respond to this revelation, Richard comments:

> I don't think you understand the reasons these people have for wanting surgery – it's not vanity or celebrity-inspired. They just don't want to look fazed at work, or appear too hassled by the demands of the job.

This is fundamental to life in the high-finance lane. Corporate pressure relies on its opposite to define its ideal image. Appearing comfortable and relaxed is vitally important to Richard, no matter what the pressure. Indeed, representations of youth, energy and vitality are what make possible the deeper control, calm and commitment of the corporate self.

The culture of the world of investment banking is thus of crucial importance in grasping Richard's experimentation with cosmetic surgery. There is an economic imperative at the heart of Richard's desire to reverse the biological clock, and to trump ageing through eradication of his mid-life belly. In this sense, Richard's turn to cosmetic surgery might be said to overturn narcissism and reinstate the primacy of economics. Yet in doing so Richard reveals that it is love of fantasy as much as economic rationalism that drives his search to outflank death and the laws of nature. The reign of narcissism promoted by the new capitalism (expressed by Richard as 'it pays to look good') is merely a mask tried on by investment bankers, one that in fact occludes their own subjection to the unfathomable powers of multinational capitalism. So it may well pay to look good, since the appearance of power is what increasingly serves to solidify power in objectified form. But even more important is Richard's recognition that power is never self-contained. 'Cosmetic surgery', he tells me, ' helps me escape from standing out – in terms of the visible distress of looking worried, or old.' Surgery assists, in short, with the corporate dilemma of high-pressed work environments. For Richard, it permits him to take such pressure in his stride.

Undergoing cosmetic surgery in order to obtain a career edge is not an altogether new social phenomenon. The historical dimensions of this social trend have been well documented by the American scholar Elizabeth Haiken. In *Venus Envy: A History of Cosmetic Surgery*, Haiken traces Americans' faith in the gospel of self-improvement through plastic surgery back to the Depression of the 1930s. With the launch of a new ethos of self-making within the broader narrative of capitalism as a result of the Depression, she argues,

> some Americans, admittedly grasping at straws, held fast to the idea that control over the limited area of physical appearance at least offered a chance for social and economic security, and that others simply acted on the belief that it couldn't hurt.[1]

It was a measure of how truly catastrophic social things became in the late 1920s and '30s that an ideology of self-improvement was launched at a cost so severe to the well-being of individuals.

For Haiken, self-preservation became all about the re-making and renewal of the body in the context of the wider economy. It is perhaps no wonder that, faced with the oppressive nature of this ideology, many surgeons also came round to such a worldview. As Haiken notes:

> Whilst surgeons continued to guard their turf, insisting that they would operate only when they, in their pro-

fessional capacity, decided a problem was significant enough to warrant surgical intervention, the new social and economic justification for cosmetic surgery persuaded them to listen to prospective patients' complaints with new sympathy.[2]

Haiken documents a broad range of human sufferings in the shape of demands for surgical interventions, all lying within the ambit of the economic field. These include the following:

Interior decorator Muriel Johnson, who as early as 1931 wondered if a face-lift would assist her to secure new clients.

Richard Thomas, a man from the 1930s seeking a new nose for career advancement.

Model Lily Pells who, in 1933, sought cosmetic surgery to correct her nose.

An English woman with two children, Jane Hatch, who in 1941 hoped a new nose would bring better career prospects.

This attempt to bridge the gap between commerce and cosmetics is, however, endorsed by Haiken only up to a point. *Venus Envy*, for all its attention to the economics of surgery, is too attentive to the intricate interplay of psychology, history and society to let the economy function as the final determinant in the rise of cosmetic surgical culture. Questions of cultural economy are thus carefully sealed off from the wider social forces they are supposed to transfigure. 'The widely held conviction', writes Haiken,

that beauty had, in the modern world, assumed a social and economic value helped to persuade surgeons to reevaluate their attitudes toward cosmetic surgery . . . But, trained and accustomed to defining their work in

113

terms of medicine, they resisted any line of reasoning that seemed to place them on a par with hairdressers and beauticians.

There is a difference, it transpires, between recognizing that surgery may contain social and economic benefits, and the view that, through surgical enhancements to the body, the individual stands to gain various resources in the wider social arena. Haiken considers the former rather than the latter standpoint, and even then the economic field appears only as an afterthought to her historical study.

Against the backdrop of the global rise of the new economy, the field of the economic can no longer be analysed as a mere 'addition' to social and historical forces governing cosmetic surgical culture. *Pace* Haiken, the sociology I develop for cosmetic surgical culture, all the way from popular media and celebrity to consumerism, globalization and work in the new economy, may look perversely unhistorical. The past half-century, however, has been a time of unprecedented economic expansion, with major booms not only in the global North but also in Asia and Australasia. To this we must add the technological revolution of recent decades, which more than any other factor has transformed the ways in which we now work and live. Yet the new economy remains shot through with a contradiction: if globalization represents an advanced stage of capitalist production and consumption, it is undoubtedly one that results in significantly greater economic inequality and social instability. Thus, as regards cosmetic surgery, the truth is that for millions of anxious or hassled workers around the world makeover culture offers not so much an opportunity to stand out from the crowd, but a chance to go *unnoticed*. It offers a respite from ageing in an ageist society; it offers a temporary escape route from the end-of-line identities that come with being past one's sell-by date. In this final chapter, developing on this theme, I wish to explore these links between globalization, the new economy and the explosion of popular interest in cosmetic surgical culture. I shall look in particular at how the increasing penetration of cosmetic surgery into daily life has altered the nature of work, employment and unemployment.

'Sometimes Nips and Tucks Can Be Career Moves', announced the *New York Times* in early 2006.[3] The link between physical attractiveness and employment advancement today, the paper's journalist Eryn Brown argued, is transforming lives, and rapidly. The emphasis is very much on career 'moves' – onwards and upwards. There can be no falling back on traditional ideas of 'careers' or 'jobs-for-life', both of which are eroding before our eyes. Work identities today, for the most part, are built out of active processes of remaking and reconstruction. If the new economy promises hi-tech jobs with stock options, short-term contracts and creative working environments, it is also inaugurates unprecedented levels of outsourcing, lay-offs, age discrimination and job insecurity.

At the centre of the story reported by the *New York Times* was Manhattan's Ginny Clark, a 62-year-old stock trader who had just undergone a face-lift. Though many of her fellow workers were preparing to retire from Wall Street as they entered their more advanced years, Clark felt no such compulsion. On the contrary, her hunger for work – for the challenges issued by economic markets – lay undiminished. But her problem was that she didn't feel she looked the part, at least not any longer. This profoundly affected her self-confidence. She was surrounded by workers many years younger; indeed, she was dating a man ten years her junior. She felt old, and increasingly outdated.

Ginny Clark seized the opportunity, consulted a surgeon about obtaining a younger look and underwent the surgeon's knife. The reason she sought cosmetic surgery, she commented, was to extend her career. As she remarked, 'cosmetic surgery gives you a leg up if you want to stick around'. The really successful people today, she thought, were the young ones. The young are winners and the old losers – consigned to retirement and the scrap heap. In such a world, Clark sought readmittance to the former club. And cosmetic surgery, she reasoned, held the key.

But it was not only Ginny Clark who subscribed to such a bleak view of the world; so did her physician, Dr Alan Matarasso. He is reported by the newspaper as summarizing the world of work thus:

> On Wall Street, most of these guys retire in their mid-40s or 50s. You have hedge fund managers who are 28 years old. So at 50, you feel old.

In this newly fashioned, postmodern world of work, what is valued today can change overnight. Nobody and nothing is valued for the long term, least of all employees. Who or what is of value to a company can change in an instant. The ideal response, in such a situation, is to emphasize your personal assets – particularly if they revolve on youth, vitality and sex appeal. It is better to promote your own assets than rely on your track record, since the latter is already yesterday's news. Or, for that matter, yesterday's track record may be out of step with today's corporate objectives. Workers need to imagine new forms of work commitment, which increasingly centre in the new economy on the capacity and willingness to undergo self-reinvention. This is what Ginny Clark had signed up to, whether she knew it or not.

Such a crisis of self-identity, and its accompanying corrective strategy of self-reinvention, finds a parallel in the *speed* of surgical procedures today. It may be the spirit of self-reinvention that counts at the level of the organization or company, but there is no makeover without sacrifice, no bodily 'improvement' without physical pain. Yet cosmetic surgical culture now offers men and women not only a route out of their present-day social and economic woes, but also a way out unnoticeably and swiftly. No wonder, then, that Brown refers to the work of Wendy Lewis, a New York consultant advising on the necessity of planning with military precision the *timing* of surgical procedures in the work schedule. Wendy Lewis, writes Brown,

> advises clients to consider carefully how they will fit an operation – or upkeep, if a client is having Botox injections or other small treatments – into their work schedules. She steers busy clients away from doctors who tend to run late on appointments, and discourages patients from undergoing complicated procedures that would keep them away from work for more than a few days.[4]

From eye tweaks and laser treatments to body lifts and nose jobs, a professional consultant is always near at hand to advise on the right surgeon and, above all else, the logistics of recovery time.

There are different ways, as we have seen, in which people are encouraged, cajoled or seduced by consumer society to consider cosmetic surgery as expanding their lifestyle horizons. But there is also a deeper set of social forces at work in the branding of cosmetic surgery as a consumer lifestyle choice. The root of the problem is largely cultural, driven by a new corporate ethos that flexible and ceaseless reinvention is the only adequate response to globalization. Clearly, globalization is a world of transformations, affecting every aspect not only of what we do but what we think about our lives. For better or worse, globalization has given rise to the 24/7 society, in which continual self-actualization and dramatic self-reinvention have become all the rage.

Globalization has become one of the crucial buzzwords of our times – and our lives in these times.[5] One needs to be careful when assessing arguments about the consequences of globalization, since what people call 'globalization' has many different meanings, not all of them coherent, few reconcilable. One central part of what globalization means for many critics is advanced capitalism in its broadest sense, and thus by implication the term has come to revolve around Americanization. This is the view that globalization is a central driver in the export of American commerce and culture, of the vast apparatus of mass consumerism, of the unleashing of us-controlled turbo-capitalism. Others view globalization through the lens of a much longer historical perspective, beginning with the age of discovery and the migrations from the Old World to the New.

A full discussion of the many facets of globalization goes beyond the scope of this book. But I do want to stay with the theme of our globalizing world for much of the discussion of this chapter, since I will go on to suggest that there are important new links between the speed and dynamism of processes of intensive globalization on the one hand and the popular explosion of interest in the makeover industries and cosmetic surgical culture on the other. In this connection, it is the impact of communications media and new information technologies that is perhaps of most importance in grasping what is truly new about globalization. Political theorist David Held captures this point well when he contends:

> What is new about the modern global system is the chronic intensification of patterns of interconnectedness mediated by such phenomena as the modern communications industry and new information technology and the spread of globalization in and through new dimensions of interconnectedness: technological, organizational, administrative and legal, among others, each with their own logic and dynamic of change.[6]

Transformations in the organizational and corporate dimensions of global interconnectedness, to anticipate my argument, are creating the conditions in which instant self-reinvention through cosmetic surgery occur.

The impact of multinational corporations, able to export industrial production to low-wage spots around the globe and to restructure investment in the West away from manufacture to the finance, service and communications sectors, has spelt major changes in the ways people live their lives and how they approach work, as well as how they position themselves within the employment marketplace. While employment has become much more complex than in previous periods as a result of the acceleration of globalization, one crucial institutional fact redefining the contemporary condition has been the rapid decline of lifetime employment. The end of a job-for-life, or of a career developed within a single organization, has been interpreted by some critics as heralding the arrival of a 'new economy' – flexible, mobile, networked. Global financier and philanthropist George Soros argues that 'transactions' now substitute for 'relationships' in the modern economy.[7] In *The Corrosion of Character*, American sociologist Richard Sennett, musing on the personal consequences of work in conditions of globalization, suggests that a

> change in modern institutional structure has accompanied short-term, contract, or episodic labor. Corporations have sought to remove layers of bureaucracy, to become flatter and more flexible organizations. In place of organizations as pyramids, management wants now to think of organizations as networks . . . This means that promotions and dismissals tend not to be based on clear, fixed rules, nor are work tasks crisply defined; the network is constantly redefining its structure.[8]

For Sennett, the rise of flexible capitalism, however much flexibility and risk-taking are said to give people more freedom to shape the direction of their lives, actually leads to crushing new burdens and oppressions. Flexible capitalism is 'flexible' only in as far as its workers and consumers accept the dictates of a post-hierarchical world, accept that it is they and they alone who must strive to be ever more flexible, and accept the abandonment of traditional models of work, as well as standard definitions of success.

Authors such as Sennett see the flexibility demanded of workers by multinational corporations as demonstrating the reality of globalization, promoting a dominant conception of individuals as dispensable and disposable. It is against this sociological backdrop that he cites statistics indicating that the average American college student graduating today can expect to hold twelve positions or jobs in their lifetime, in addition to which they will be required to change their skills base at least three times. From this viewpoint, yesteryear's job-for-life is replaced today by short-term contract work. No wonder flexible capitalism has its discontents, who find to their dismay that the alleged benefits of free markets are less and less apparent. In a subsequent work, *The Culture of the New Capitalism*, Sennett spells out the deeper emotional consequences of such big organizational changes thus: 'people fear being displaced, sidelined, or underused. The institutional model of the future does not furnish them a life narrative at work, or the promise of much security in the public realm.'[9] Today's corporate culture of short-termism is producing a thorough-going erosion of the loyalty and trust that employees vest in their workplaces. 'Work identities', writes Sennett, 'get used up, they become exhausted, when institutions themselves are continually reinvented.'[10] In a corporate world where people are always thinking about their next career move, or preparing for major change, it is very difficult to remain loyal – and ultimately dysfunctional – to any one company or organization.

In this regard, the speed of change unleashed by the global electronic economy – and particularly the impact of institutional change on our working and private lives – is critical. In 2006 Princeton economist Gene Grossman identified a new stage of globalization, one that centres on the virtually instant transfer of service jobs to low-wage economies.[11] He argues that this 'global electronic off-shoring' is fast changing our ways of living and working – and will continue to do so in dramatic ways over the coming years. For Grossman, electronic offshoring refers to more than the rise of call centres in countries such as India. For any service job can be electronically outsourced if it involves substantial reliance on information technology and involves little face-to-face interaction. And this is the really dramatic part of Grossman's research: he estimates that in the near future no fewer than 30–40 million service jobs in the US will become open to electronic offshoring.

Clearly, if Grossman is right, this spells major change not only for the US but more broadly for the global North. Work-ers throughout the service sectors of the expensive cites of the West, as with manufacturing some decades previously, will be exposed to intense competition from overseas as never before. And not just unskilled or semi-skilled workers are at risk. The highly skilled and highly educated – working in finance, legal, medical and hi-tech sectors – are also threatened. This, Grossman suggests, will have traumatic consequences for individual identities and local communities, especially as regards the provision of economic and emo-tional support for the many whose livelihoods are threat-ened. Where does this leave people in terms of their work? Consigned to the spectre of uselessness? Not necessarily, thankfully. For one thing, retraining and redeployment are now crucial offshoots of many large-scale organizational re-trenchments. Moreover, offshoring to date has affected only a small proportion of jobs in the advanced economies, and it's not possible to say with any degree of confidence how the global job market will develop in the future. But whilst this may be reassuring in one sense, it clearly isn't in another. How could anyone now believe, say, in the long-term management of companies or organizations, or for that matter in long-term careers, after reading Grossman? Dilemmas and quandaries are now the plight of contemporary women and men seeking to sketch out a basically safe psychological platform when moving from job to job, contract to contract, network to network. But in our fast globalizing electronic economy, the more astute accept that short-term jobs, contracts and networks are the new realities. What matters is flexibility – the plastic, reshaped sense of self that these new institutional forms of the global economy at once produce and demand. Thus the typical modern dilemma: how to be flexible enough to survive high levels of personal and cultural drift without being left drained of identity.

It is, to be sure, a profound and anxiety-provoking set of socio-economic changes. The fast, short-term, techy culture of globalization is unleashing – I am suggesting – a new paradigm of self-making. In a world of short-term contracts, endless downsizings, just-in-time deliveries and multiple careers, the capacity to change and reinvent oneself has become fundamental. A faith in flexibility, plasticity and incessant reinvention – all this means we are no longer judged on what we have done and achieved; we're now judged on our flexibility, on our readiness for personal makeover.

How is this brave new world of short-termism affecting our sense of identity? And in what ways does the new economy disrupt and disturb the ways in which work and employment have long been cast? Sociologist Zygmunt Bauman provides some useful leads in this connection, particularly in his contention that an increasingly liquid world renders identity oppressive by the very superficiality of its fictions of instant change. In his provocative book *Wasted Lives*, Bauman contends that the central anxiety of the twenty-first century is that of the fear of disposability. This is the fear people today have of being dumped, displaced and discarded. 'What we all seem to fear', writes Bauman,

> is abandonment, exclusion, being rejected, blackballed, disowned, dropped, stripped of what we are, being refused what we wish to be. We fear being left alone, helpless and hapless. Barred company, loving hearts and helping hands. We fear to be dumped – our turn for the scrapyard. What we miss most badly is the certainty that all that won't happen – not to us. We miss exemption – from the universal and ubiquitous threat of exemption. We dream of immunity against the toxic effluvia of refuse tips.[12]

For Bauman, the institutional changes spawned by globalization, high technology and the new economy have given rise to a fluid life – a 'liquid modernity', as he aptly puts it – that spells the end of thinking long-term. Liquid life, says Bauman, is lived under the anxious shadow of globalization; it is a precarious life, in which individuals try to figure out how to 'keep up' with the social conditions of constant uncertainty bred by global finance. As Bauman puts it,

> There are the seemingly random, haphazard and utterly unpredictable moves and shifts and drifts of what for the lack of a more precise name are called 'forces of globalization'. . . They change beyond recognition, and without warning, the familiar landscapes and cityscapes where the anchors of our durable and reliable security used to be cast. They reshuffle people and play havoc with their social identities.[13]

The havoc in question concerns the erosion of people's ability to manage long-term relationships, let alone think about possible trajectories of the self in the longer term. What Bauman wants to highlight are the insidious ways in which global capitalism penetrates daily life, reorganizing the structures of working life and corporate culture. For better or for worse, many companies – he contends – have responded to the widespread erosion of trust between capital and labour, between management and workers, by pushing their employees to adopt more flexible identity strategies in order to maximize their profits. The gas giant Enron, he argues, is a good example of this. Long before the infamous corruption scandal that projected Enron to front-page news in the early 2000s, the company had pioneered an employee review system in which 15 per cent of their workforce was ritually retrenched twice a year, with a warning issued to 30 per cent to lift their performance. As Bauman points out,

> this was not a matter of a one-off test – life in Enron was a day-in, day-out test, the pressure never relenting. No credit of trust accrued, the memory of the most impressive success would hardly survive to the next morning unless yesterday's 'killing' was followed by another, yet more dazzling.[14]

A sense of self that is orientated to the short term was consequently produced, in which past experience and accumulated talent or skill counted for little, if anything. 'Enron', writes Bauman,

> was not a plot on which to build lifelong plans: just a camping site for portable tents easy to pitch and easier yet to fold. Life in the company constantly hovered on the brink of redundancy and felt like a daily rehearsal of waste disposal. Everyone's turn to be disposed of was never far away, and so by the time it arrived it could be greeted in most cases as a welcome relief of tension rather than a random blow of fate.[15]

Whilst it is arguably the case that the kind of managerial practice and organizational attitude to employees that Bauman underscores in discussing Enron is somewhat extreme, such ideologies of flexible self-making and reinvention are increasingly on the rise across institutions in the private and public sectors. Moreover, his account of liquid life is one that obviously chimes nicely with a globalized world of increased mobility, technological revolution and instant communication. Yet whatever the adequacy of this social theory of liquidity for grasping contemporary social change,[16] I do want to argue that Bauman's contention concerning fear of disposability sheds light on the new social forces motivating people to demand instant self-reinvention through the makeover industries and surgical culture.

In *The New Individualism*, the American sociologist Charles Lemert and I argued that, throughout the polished, expensive cities of the West, there was an emergent 'new individualism' built upon continual self-actualization and instant self-reinvention. This is nowhere more evident today, we argued, than in the pressure consumerism puts on us to 'transform' and 'improve' every aspect of ourselves: not just our homes and gardens but also our careers, our food, our clothes, our sex lives, our faces, minds and bodies. This reinvention trend occurs all around us, not only in the rise of DIY and the instant identity makeovers of reality TV, but also in compulsive consumerism, speed dating and therapy culture. In a world that places a premium on instant gratification, the desire for immediate results has never been as pervasive or acute. We have become accustomed to emailing others across the planet in seconds, buying flashy consumer goods with the click of a mouse and drifting in and out of relations with others without long-term commitments. Is it any wonder that we now have different expectations about life's possibilities and the potential for change?

The privatization of all things social is crucial to this. In the new economy, our language for expressing individualism is more and more fixed into the syntax of possession, ownership, control and market value. Ownership of the self as an asset becomes fundamental to the movements and choices of those with unfixed identities in wider economy; this is a fertile form of self-assertion in an economy given over to ceaseless marketing, advertising and branding. Have no fixed identity, and will reinvent! This is the catch-cry of today's new economy. Yet the consequences of today's instant self-reinvention go further down than just our working lives. The ceaselessly reinventing worker of today does not shift from a negative to a positive identity in the act of self-transformation; the reinvention craze is desperation incarnate. This is a neurotic, tragic creed that flows from the constant uncertainties of the new economy. Consequently, what we witness today is a form of individualism based on a new cultural imperative for people to be more efficient, faster, leaner, inventive and self-actualizing than they were previously – not sporadically, but day-in, day-out. Such an imperative lends to social life a radically experimental quality, with the thrills and spills of personal experiments to the fore. But the emotional costs are also high; many of the stories we recount of contemporary women and men in *The New Individualism* are those of personal confusion, intense anxiety and disquieting depression. Such emotional tribulations are not simply private problems, however, because the new individualism is first and foremost a consequence of our world of intensive globalization. In smashing apart traditional national boundaries, globalization, ironically, offers people a kind of 'absolute freedom' to do whatever they like. The irony is that the world of 'everything goes' has become crippling, as the anxiety of choice floats unhinged from both practical and ethical considerations as to what is worth pursuing. For those enticed and seduced by the new individualism, the danger of self-reinvention is a form of change so rapid and so complete that identity becomes disposable. Instead of finding ourselves, we lose ourselves.

Many people are opting for personal makeover or cosmetic surgery in a bid to improve their chances of keeping up with the intense economic changes wrought by globalization. One professional woman I interviewed, for example, felt that her surgical 'touch-up' had given her a significant edge over competitors within her company, improving her prospects of remaining on the senior management team. Surgery appears here as a strategy to keep in the game, or to stay one step ahead. It is against this backdrop that the notion of 'making the cut' starts to take on quite particular personal and organizational ramifications.

Dr Ronald Iverson, an expert on cosmetic surgery and one-time chairman of the public education committee for the American Society of Plastic and Reconstructive Surgeons, commented as early as 1991 that the rapid rise in the number of men opting for surgery had been driven, above all, by the possibility of improved job prospects. Older men and especially executives, he explained to the *Wall Street Journal*, were 'competing with younger people to get back in the workplace'.[17] Trying to compete in such a market through reliance only on one's previous achievements, the reader quickly discerns, is considered an arduous, soul-destroying experience. This is especially the case for those executives who look 'tired', who may have let themselves 'go', or were no longer up for demonstrating their willingness to be disciplined, fit, energetic, self-inventive and so on. In our society of instant self-reinvention, cosmetic surgery offers such men a way forward – or, so readers of the *Wall Street Journal* were informed. Cosmetic surgery is not just for neurotic narcissists. 'Doctors and patients call it an investment for the future, like a college degree or a new business suit.' Yet there are risks – both cosmetic and commercial consequences that one doesn't know and cannot anticipate. 'Cosmetic surgery is not a panacea and will not guarantee anyone a better chance at a job.'

The fact that one has undergone the surgeon's knife may not give you carte blanche to relaunch your career however you may choose; but it does provide many people – according to contemporary media reports – with a second chance in work and employment. London's *Financial Times*, for example, ran the following story on how cosmetic surgery may combat age discrimination in the workplace or boost a flagging career – citing some of these cases:

> A vice-president who, at the age of sixty, was retrenched. Unable to find a new position, and convinced that he was being discriminated against because of his older appearance, he underwent a face-lift. He was appointed to a new vice-presidential position in a large company two months following the surgery.

> A fifty year old Californian salesman, who was discriminated against at work because bags under his eyes made him look exhausted. Management thought this might be the result of a drinking problem, and he was told to go on holiday. Instead, he has the bags surgically removed, and was consequently promoted.

> A forty-five year old female executive in California, who felt that her authority within the company was being eroded by an energetic younger woman. After the executive underwent procedures for a facelift and eye surgery, the younger woman ceased to pose a threat.

Cosmetic surgery is, for the most part, presented in such wildly transformative terms throughout the *Financial Times* article. However, there are also words of caution. It all depends, the reader is told, on how frequently cosmetic procedures are carried out. Surgery may be an act of self-transformation, but it requires some degree of restraint.

'Don't be too ambitious. Two or three facelifts may help you look younger. Five will make you look odd.'[18]

The employment remedy offered by cosmetic surgery may need to be administered in small doses, but there can be no doubting the sheer scale of the makeover industries today. Nor, it seems, the escalating and widespread viewpoint that an individual's working life can flourish under conditions of surgically enhanced beauty. In a subsequent article printed some years after the story I've mentioned above, the *Financial Times* announced: 'cosmetic "enhancements" and beauty [are] now linked to professional success'.[19] The people interviewed on this occasion by the *Financial Times* lived in Spain, where it was found that 'professional women and a growing number of men are turning to cosmetic surgery to boost their self-esteem and their careers'. Indeed, employment, skills and working patterns in Spain have been transformed as a consequence of the country's love affair with artificially enhanced bodies. According to the International Society of Aesthetic Plastic Surgeons, Spain ranked sixth out of forty-three countries surveyed for its volume of surgical procedures – behind the USA, Canada, Mexico, Brazil and Argentina. And not only was cosmetic surgery understood as influencing employment and work behaviour in the new economy in Spain, it also comprised an increasingly large stake of the new capitalism itself. Corporacion Dermoestetica, Spain's largest cosmetic surgery group, with clinics in the UK, Italy and Portugal, floated on the Spanish stock exchange – the subject of the FT article.

The connections between cosmetics and commerce operate, however, within a framework of cultural influence on other levels too. To grasp the hold that cosmetic surgical culture now exerts in business environments, we need to keep in mind the reflexive, or endlessly circular, nature of media information today. A good example of this was the widely reported UK survey, from 2005, that more than a quarter of women executives would consider cosmetic surgery in order to improve their career prospects. 'The research reveals', reported M2 *Presswire*,

> that more than a quarter of female executives would be prepared to go under the knife if they thought it would get them ahead in business. Such is women's preoccupation with their physical appearance that 26 per cent would consider a face-lift, 27 per cent plastic surgery and 28 per cent Botox treatments if they thought it would boost their career prospects.[20]

In addition to which, less invasive procedures were almost universally endorsed by those interviewed.

Little surprise here, one might think. After all, we have come to expect a society like ours, so attuned to the ethos of self-reinvention, to support cosmetic surgical culture at every step. But the reader of this M2 *Presswire* report may note that this 'influential survey' was carried out by the Aziz Corporation – one of the UK's leading independent communications consultancies. The charter of the Aziz Corporation, as it happens, is to 'add value to businesses by ensuring their people are effective communicators'. As a sociologist, I am struck by the possible double loop, or circularity, of information at play here. A survey that uncovers social trends on the 'opening up' of people's attitudes to the uses of cosmetic surgery to advance their careers is carried out by a communications consultancy that, in turn, advises businesses on employees' image development and presentation skills. This is where the cultural links between cosmetics and commerce are most theatrical or performative. In the new economy, business participation in (and adoption of the strategies of) cosmetic surgical culture requires a certain kind of rhetoric. Consultants, image advisers, life coaches and the so-called creative industries all testify to the performative dimensions of cosmetic surgical culture.

In the contemporary age, the combined institutional formula of globalization, high technology and the new economy has given rise to widespread fears about being made redundant. Like fear in general, this specific fear of disposability, a 'wasted life' in the apt phrase of Bauman, is both positive and negative, self-generative and self-destructive. If there is something constructive about today's disposability fears it is not only because they propel people into a more active engagement with their lives, but also because they help generate novel forms of self-experimentation and personal transformation. It is not hard to see the bearing of the instabilities of global finance on people's decisions to return to university for a second degree, or seek retraining or re-skilling as a means of realizing the contemplated career move. It is perhaps more of a stretch to see the vagaries of global finance as the ground or prop that supports experiments in life coaching, on-line therapy or cosmetic surgery. Yet as far as today's cultural obsession with cosmetic surgery goes at any rate, I have been suggesting that a blend of economic and psychological factors does indeed shape people's fears of disposability and about being made redundant. The vulnerable need to reconstruct the self – to rebuild the working life from without and within – is what also gives rise to the crazed excess of cosmetic surgical culture. It is perhaps the indiscriminate indifference of the global economy that results in a self-violence of surgical alterations and bodily transpositions as an imagined strategy in which people seek to keep pace, or even outflank, the logic of business and the marketplace. As we will now consider in greater depth, such self-violence is driven largely by the cultural value placed on youth, sex and beauty.

I want now to broaden this account to suggest that cosmetic surgical culture – driven largely by fear of disposability in our age of intensive globalization – works as a *screen* onto which people project their discontent. I want to suggest, too, that people increasingly turn to cosmetic surgery when socio-economic circumstances link deeply with *melancholic* aspects of identity. Melancholia, as Freud uncovered, is a form of intense sadness over nothing in particular. It is a kind of free-floating grief that attaches to various persons, objects and events – from the death of a loved one to the assassination of a political leader to the break-up of a pop group. A distinctive feature of melancholic experience is the manner in which it locks the self in relation to others and the wider world; this involves emotional fixation and the closing down of human complexity. The discontented husband who refuses to admit the desirability of his wife because she is now 'middle-aged'. The older woman who buys endless trend fashions she will never wear for fear of looking foolish in a youth-obsessed culture. The ageing executive who resorts to cosmetic practices or surgery as a means of competing with his younger and energetic colleagues. All are melancholic identities.

Psychoanalysis gives useful leads on what is going on here. The relentless preoccupation with loss in various versions of psychoanalysis concerns both the *fear* and the *pain* of loss. From Freud to Melanie Klein to Julia Kristeva, the individual forges a relation to itself and other people through loss: the loss of loved ones, the loss of selves, the loss of pasts. When thinking of loss from a psychoanalytic point of view, it is necessary to stress therefore that people create themselves through forgetting and remembering their losses. In what follows, I want to look at psychoanalytic theory in a little detail to consider how loss operates within the broader contours of cosmetic surgical culture.

From his earliest writings, Freud argued that self-experience begins with the experience of loss. The mother (or primary caretaker) is for Freud the child's first and most significant loss. Through her absence, the infant comes to recognize that mother is different from itself. For it is only through the mother's absence, says Freud, that the infant comes to desire her presence. This founding moment of separation is both frightening and exciting, and in order to cope the infant creates fantasies about the mother as a compensation for her painful absence. In other words, the infant reacts to the absence of the mother in reality by imagining her present in fantasy. In its capacity for imagination, writes Freud, the infant has 'created an object out of the mother'.[21]

It is worth considering what the denial of loss might mean at the level of the inner world, given the emphasis on repression in psychoanalysis. In his essay of 1915, 'Mourning and Melancholia', Freud reconstructs the connections between love and loss on the one hand, and the limits of identification and identity on the other. 'The loss of a love object', he writes 'is an excellent opportunity for the ambivalence in love-relationships to make itself effective and come into the open'.[22] The loss of a loved person, he suggests, brings into play ambivalence and aggression. Under such circumstances, both one's passion and one's anger for lost love comes to the fore. Since the other person is loved, the self incorporates some aspect of the loved other into itself in order to maintain the emotional tie. But because the other person is also hated, this incorporated aspect of the other now becomes something despised within the self.

On this basis, Freud distinguishes between 'normal mourning' and the 'complex of melancholia'. Freud considers mourning a normal response to the loss of a loved person. In 'normal mourning', the self incorporates aspects of the other person and then gradually detaches itself from the lost love. By acknowledging the pain of absence, the mourner draws emotionally from the lost love; he or she borrows, as it were, personality traits and feelings associated with the loved person, and in so doing is able to work through these feelings of loss. In the 'complex of melancholia', the individual fails to break from the lost love, keeping hold of the object through identification. Unable to mourn, the melancholic cannot express love and hate directly towards the lost love, and instead denigrates its own ego. Freud describes this melancholic process as an 'open wound': the melancholic is caught in a spiralling of identifications, a spiralling in which hatred rounds back upon the self, 'emptying the ego until it is totally impoverished'. Whereas the mourner gradually accepts that the lost love no longer exists, the melancholic engages in denial in order to protect the self from loss.

Another way of putting all this is to say that selfhood is drafted against the backdrop of our willingness or unwillingness to mourn loss. If the pain of loss can be tolerated, the individual subject can set about relinquishing primary involvements. If the pain of loss cannot be tolerated, there is a grafting of sadness on to the lost object itself, a reaction that transforms mourning into melancholia.[23] Language plays a central role here. Words, for Freud, are the means to figure out loss. Language fills in for what has been lost. Words are a stop gap, helping to close up the pain of lost love.[24] 'The child', writes Julia Kristeva,

> becomes irredeemably sad before uttering his first words: this is because he has been irrevocably, desperately separated from the mother, a loss that causes him to try to find her again, along with other objects of love, first in the imagination, then in words.[25]

By invoking psychoanalytic theory to consider the complexities of the relation between self, loss and melancholia, my objective is to raise fresh questions as to how we might think about the grief that cosmetic surgical culture both contains and represses. In doing so, I want to focus on an aspect of the debate over cosmetic surgery that is perhaps not very familiar. This is an argument about the emerging global economy of grief in these early days of the twenty-first century.

The idea that cosmetic surgical culture both contains and represses melancholic grief raises the following questions.

In what ways does loss manifest itself in cosmetic surgical culture? How does an unconscious refusal to work through loss – the hallmark of melancholia – attach itself to the lures of beauty enhancement or body augmentation? If the short-termism of surgical solutions is now a culturally sanctioned means of displacing the power of loss in our lives, what are the longer-term consequences of such human decisions?

Just as flexible capitalism engages in ceaseless organizational restructurings, so now do people – employees, employers, consumers. Don DeLillo argues that global capitalism generates transformations at 'the speed of light', not only in terms of the sudden movement of factories, the mass migration of workers and the instant shifts of liquid capital, but in 'everything from architecture to leisure time to the way people eat and sleep and dream'.[26] In thinking about the complex ways in which our emotional lives are altered by the socio-economic changes wrought by globalization, I want to add to the wealth of transformations mentioned by DeLillo by focusing on people's changing experiences of their bodies as a result of new cosmetic surgical technologies. My argument is that global forces, in transforming economic and technological structures, penetrate to the very tissue of our personal and emotional lives.

Most writers agree that globalization involves the dramatic rewriting of national and local boundaries. The overnight shifts of capital investment, the transnational spread of multipurpose production, the privatization of government-owned institutions, the endless remodellings of finance, the rise of new technologies and the unstable energy of 24/7 stock markets: such images of multinational capitalism bring starkly into focus the extent to which today's world is being remade, and daily. I have been suggesting that such changes seep deeply into daily life, and are affecting greater and greater numbers of people. The values of the new global economy are increasingly being adopted by people to remodel their lives. The emphasis is on living the short-term contract lifestyle (from what one wears to where one lives to how one works), of ceaseless cosmetic transformations and bodily improvements, of instant metamorphosis and multiple identities.

A growing faith in dismantling, deconstructing and destabilizing existing institutional structures is now echoed in private life, and perhaps nowhere more so than in cosmetic surgical culture. The power of endless self-reinvention strenuously advocated by the makeover industries touches not only on fears that people experience about being made redundant or rendered disposable, but also on anxieties over youth and its passing, time and its dissolution, as well as ageing and the ultimate constraint of death.

The first way in which cosmetic surgical culture calls grief into play is through the relentless stress placed on youth in modern societies. Of course, this is not entirely new: youth, as interwoven with representations of sex and beauty, has long formed part of the cultural obsessions and ideals of the West. Today, however, we witness a far denser media and informational system of diffusing images, signs and symbols pertaining to youth. This cultural worship of youth at once renders young bodies as desirable and older bodies as not. A certain self-awareness about and understanding of bodies has thus been increasingly generalized in a startlingly new way. Among populations of the pricey cities of the West, the body is now an immensely fashionable concern – certainly the youthful, sleek, verging on anorexic, body, not the older one.

This is where cosmetic surgical culture comes into its own. By drawing attention to the visible signs of ageing, from blotchy patches to crow's feet, the makeover industries attempt to 'sell youth' to an ageist culture. From the skin tightening of mini-face-lifts to the enhancements of collagen, cosmetic surgeons and the makeover industries seek to sell their 'products' through associations with youth. But what is considered youthful appears to be getting ever younger. As Shelley Gare writes,

> cosmetic surgeons now proudly say there have been so many improvements and breakthroughs in their procedures, women can start having rejuvenation treatments in their 30s. We may be trying to believe 50 is the new 30, but with such emphasis on looks, lines and reinvention, 30 is in danger of eventually looking like the new 100.[27]

It is not difficult to see in all this the influence of grief, the hungering for lost youth, combined with the attempt to outflank the pain of loss through cosmetic procedures and surgical interventions.

A second sign of the imprint of grief in cosmetic surgical culture lies in its attempted freezing of time. As we enter the epoch of advanced globalization, cosmetic surgical culture has come to stand for the annihilation of time. As such, cosmetic surgery is anti-linear; it warps traditional assumptions that one starts to look older as one ages. The makeover industries thus claim to provide a glimpse of 'for-ever', the promise to arrest our biologically ageing bodies – which is to say that it is not hard to detect a good deal of wish fulfilment operating here. But if cosmetic surgical culture confers on its subjects a kind of pseudo-halt to time and ageing, it also strikes the world traumatically empty of movement, development, progression. 'The economic and symbolic value of youthful bodies', writes Margaret Gibson,

> creates a false but nevertheless seductive fantasy of bodies as static and unchanging. Frozen in time through the image, the youthful and beautiful are idealized as eternal forms appearing to defy, or, alternatively, not appearing to embody, temporal mortal existence.[28]

But if this alleged arresting of time in cosmetic surgical culture has a soothing, compensatory dimension, it also has a more intimidating one. This contradiction is not accidental, since it must resort to invocations of shock, trauma and horror in order to provide the fleeting moments of imaged escape offered through the 'rewind' of age. In *Powers of Horror*, Julia Kristeva describes such horror as the realm of 'abjection'.[29] Abjection is a kind of imagined disintegration of the body in the wider frame of relations with others; it is associated by Kristeva with the ultimate imprint of the death drive, a primordial anguish or fear of a horrifying void. From this angle, the promised 'rewind' to youth offered by cosmetic surgical culture offers some sort of fantasy compensation to the horror of the void or blank that constitutes death for the unconscious. Yet this compensation remains illusory, fantasmatic. At the deeper level of emotional life – the life of the unconscious – the forces of life and death remain intricately entangled. No amount of collagen, liposuction or Botox will work to erase the deathly constituent of all human existence. The individual self, said Freud, is constituted to its roots by a primary masochism, the imprint of the death drive incarnate; this deathly form of self-destruction is what leads people to attack their lives symbolically, to annihilate the self. Cosmetic surgical culture is a fast-emerging twenty-first strategy of turning this instinct outwards. However much people attempt self-reinvention or instant makeovers, the pain of loss reappears whenever a spacing or hiatus of meaning announces itself in the psyche. This may come in the form of noticing a new ageing line, or simply less energy. In this emotional realm, there lies pain, fear, anguish.

The third sign of the containment and repression of grief in cosmetic surgical culture lies in the negation of death. Nothing reveals the ultimate uncontrollability of our lives more powerfully than death – which is one reason why countless millions have responded to the terrors of non-being by trying to organize their lives in terms of firm blueprints, fixed meanings and secure projects. 'To give death a certain kind of purity', wrote Maurice Blanchot, 'was always the task of culture: to render it authentic, personal, proper'.[30] It is the job of culture, in other words, to help rescue us from the terrors of death. Culture both structures social practices and rituals relating to mortality and suppresses our awareness of the frail character of such meaning. But as with individual psychopathology, so too cultures can develop neurotic styles of handling impending death and non-being. One crucial way in which cultural attitudes to death become bent out of shape or neurotic is through a process that sociologists call 'sequestration'.[31] The sequestration of death involves the squeezing of non-being to the sidelines of social experience. This is, in short, death displaced, denied and disowned. In our own time, one of the most graphic illustrations of this sequestration of death occurs through the transformation of dying from a community affair into a medical process. In *A Social History of Dying*, Allan Kellehear argues that we witness throughout the West today 'the disintegration of dying'. From people dying of AIDS or poverty to those in concentration camps, death is 'removed' from the wider social radar and circumscribed to a narrow institutional definition involving end-of-line medical supervision. This is perhaps nowhere more obvious today than in nursing homes, where dying has become increasingly unconnected from its biological, psychological and interpersonal roots. 'Large proportions of our dying', writes Kellehear, 'are now commonly hidden away from our communities. We do not easily witness the massive number of dying in nursing homes, in developing countries, or in totalitarian moments of our recent history.'[32]

Another contemporary Western strategy, by contrast, has involved a morbid fascination with death itself. From mangled bodies to mediated mass killings, from the medicalization of dying to the 'snuff' movies of hardcore porn: death obsesses the contemporary imagination. This may sound paradoxical, and in a certain sense it is. On the one hand, Western culture seeks to render death invisible through sequestrating it from daily life, and on the other hand it immerses itself morbidly in images and media representations of destruction, dying and death. From another angle, this contradiction is not what it at first sight seems once it is borne in mind that those caught up in such a neurotic fix are, in fact, attempting to outflank death by the deft strategy of incorporating non-being into the very tissue of life itself. To this end, it may be the case that the Freudian death drive exerts its sway. As Terry Eagleton reflects on current Western attitudes to death:

> We have to find a way of living with non-being without being in love with it, since being in love with it is the duplicitous work of the death drive. It is the death drive which cajoles us into tearing ourselves apart in order to achieve the absolute security of nothingness. Non-being is the ultimate purity. It has the unblemishedness of all negation, the perfection of a blank page.[33]

What might such morbid attempts to outwit death have to do with cosmetic surgery? My argument, following from Eagleton, is that cosmetic surgical culture today promises precisely the 'perfection of a blank page'. Both cosmetic and surgical kinds of makeover are in their different ways denials of death. In the case of Western culture, which actively devalues older people and especially older women's bodies, this denial takes the form of an imagined rewind to the splendours of youth. In rejecting mortality and the ultimate non-being of death, cosmetic surgical culture contains our aggression – the force of the death drive – only by turning it against ourselves and our bodies. What we find in invasive cosmetic surgical techniques, I am suggesting, is the corollary of a new global economy of grief. It marks the historical point in which death-avoidance is intensified. Cosmetic surgical culture represents, in Eagleton's terms, 'tearing ourselves apart in order to achieve the absolute security of nothingness'.

Summer 2007, and a typical English day looked set to unfold: overcast and grey. Staying in London with friends, I awoke very early (one of the confusions of jetlag) and set off to the Tube to catch a connection to Milton Keynes – where I was working at the Open University throughout June as a visiting professor. Later that day, I was scheduled to meet Richard Daley for our final interview.

Yet on the grey summer's morning in London, something was to happen – I was to learn of developments in the world – that would profoundly overshadow my work, as well as my final meeting with Daley. Standing at the platform at 6.30 and with time to spare, I bought the morning newspaper. Reading the headline, I read, and then re-read, the lead article – attempting to make some sense out of news that was incomprehensible.

'Dad held as girl, 2, has skull smashed', read the headline.[31] The father in question, Alberto Izaga, was a 36-year-old insurance chief who worked for Swiss Re. Police were called to the Izagas' luxury apartment near the Houses of Parliament after neighbours heard the sounds of a man and woman shouting, and a child screaming. What police discovered on entering the apartment was horrific: the Izagas' daughter, Yanire, had been punched, kicked and had her head battered against the floor by her father. She had been subsequently taken to hospital with a shattered skull and brain injuries. Several days later she died. Her father, Alberto, was sectioned under the Mental Health Act.

As I stood at the Tube trying to grasp London's latest news, and feeling completely overwhelmed by the horrendous injuries sustained by little Yanire, I noticed various details offered by the newspaper about Alberto Izaga's lifestyle and work that – within the 'story' – remained unconnected, but nonetheless seemed very relevant. Alberto, the article pointed out, was Head of Life and Health Products at Swiss Re, a company with an annual turnover of approximately £13 billion and almost 9,000 staff across thirty countries. Izaga, it transpired, was a new individualist to the core: a man of continual change, reinvention, dynamism. But he was, above all, a man under huge business pressures, experiencing severe personal strain. The newspaper article noted these aspects of Izaga's life, focusing for the most part on his stunning business success – particularly of how swiftly he had risen to the top of his profession. The high-flying Izaga's apartment was reportedly worth up to £3 million, such was its majestic views across the River Thames. He worked in the distinctive Gherkin building in the City of London, though regularly travelled abroad. A financial journalist, who had met Izaga on numerous occasions, commented:

> At the level in which he works the pressure is enormous. They all work from early morning to very late at night. They travel a lot and every decision has to be the right one. You can see people under that much pressure suddenly flipping but Alberto seemed so normal.[34]

I was struck by the sentence 'every decision has to be the right one'. I had heard this before. Modern women and men, at least those held in thrall to ideas of instant self-reinvention and personal transformation, were revolting against inherited traditions of the past, and taking a more active role in the decision-making of their lives. To get ahead, to be a player, to be promoted – active decisions were required, and they needed to be the right decisions. The right decisions about business, strategy, appearance, the future. I realized just where I had come across this mode of thinking. I had heard this in interviews with patients undergoing cosmetic surgery: 'in my profession it's all about instant impressions, and so the right appearance is crucial for confidence in decision-making'; 'it pays to look good as customers associate this with making the best decisions for them'; 'society sides with youthful and energetic people as the best custodians for making the right decisions'. I had heard it too from surgeons and practitioners. Many had depicted a clientele protective of their professional careers, eager to preserve their status and therefore hell-bent on making the 'right decisions' – of surgical procedure, of the best surgeon, of when to take time away from work, and so on and so forth.

What's peculiar about the desire for certainty in these radically different contexts – one involving psychotic breakdown and murder, the other cosmetic surgical alterations of the body – is the relentless underlining of it in global socio-economic conditions of increasing instability. Alberto Izaga was both a successful and a deranged man. The flexible behavior demanded of him by global capitalism came at the severest of costs: personal confusion, breakdown, psychotic acting-out, murder. Fortunately, what is missing when we turn to consider cosmetic surgical culture is any direct injury to others – outside the risks that a patient takes as regards their own health and life. But still I wonder, what are the emotional costs of that heady cocktail of globalization, high technology and the new economy that leads so many women and men to 'decide' to undergo the surgeon's knife? What levels of aggression, fury, rage and self-violence are unleashed here? Certainly, on the surface of it, nothing on the scale or intensity of an Alberto Izaga. In his psychotic attack upon his defenceless two-year-old daughter, Izaga crushed and destroyed the one person (and along with her, his wife) he was said to care for above all else. If the pressures of global capitalism played any role in this, as media speculation suggested it might, this could be interpreted as the desperate attempt of a man to strike the world empty of meaning. To destroy all.

It might be said that today's technologies of self-discovery are never too far from negation – the emptying out of meaning from self and world. Or, in another sense, we might say that an affinity between creation and destruction, ecstasy and excess, is peculiarly relevant to the self-reinvention of our times. What makes for makeover also makes for malevolence, and curiously it is precisely such aggression turned back on the self that comes to the fore in my final meeting with Richard Daley.

At the end of a long day of research seminars, and after travelling back from Milton Keynes to London, I sit opposite Daley for our last meeting in his plush office. At once morally conservative and economically reckless, Daley lurches from lamenting the ethical decline of society to telling me of his recent investment killings. His talk about his economic prowess has also set him, evidently, to thinking about his cosmetic surgery and how it has improved his standing at work. 'I've been widely seen as much more energetic, powerful and determined since the makeover', Daley declares to me. Since undertaking the stomach lipo, he says he's become a total convert to surgery. Like many of his peers, though, cosmetic surgery is not something Daley would easily admit to having undergone; but, privately, he acknowledges it's changed everything in his life.

Daley shows little, if any, appreciation of the limits of change. He treats personal makeover as on a par with business risk-taking, and both are ultimately concerned with advancing his career and financial standing. Yet his moral conservatism does permit, at least, some grasp of the aggression and violence that govern human affairs. He tells me he despairs of the progressive politics of Britain's New Labour and their audit culture; he sees the War on Terror as an attempt to deal with a bunch of crazed religious zealots; and, as for sexuality and post-feminism, he says that most women he meets today are just out to 'tear a man down'. If these bleak socio-political views cut across his highly calibrated optimism for personal makeover and the global economy, they do so only in a marginal sense because, ultimately, he keeps these broader fears in check or isolation. Surprisingly and unexpectedly, he then mentions the Izaga case. Perhaps not surprising that he does, since it is the talk of London. 'A terrible business', he says. The room goes quiet. I realize our time for discussion has almost come to an end. Suddenly, Daley brightens and tells me he's planning more cosmetic surgery – some further minor procedures, and possibly a mini-face-lift next year. The sudden shift away from the news of Izaga's murder of his daughter is jarring to me. As I bid Daley farewell, I leave wondering about the emotional costs of his incessant desire for change.

But Daley is far from alone in his experiments with cosmetic surgical culture. Not all that long ago, anyone who wanted cosmetic surgery would have been recommended therapy in the first instance. Today, by contrast, there is a widespread acceptance that cosmetic surgical culture is beneficial and even desirable. Especially for tough-minded, highly motivated professionals, to be surgically 'freshened up' provides an edge in the marketplace. This social transformation has not been heralded by a shift in psychological understanding. It is, rather, symptomatic of a pervasive addiction to the ethos of instant self-reinvention. And the flipside of today's reinvention craze is fear of personal disposability. For those seduced by the promises of the makeover industry, the danger of cosmetic surgery is a form of change so rapid and so complete that identity becomes disposable. The wider social costs mean that we are all debased by this soulless surgical culture.

References

Introduction

1 The survey was undertaken for *Grazia* magazine in 2005. The survey also found that a quarter of teenage boys thought they would need cosmetic surgery at some point, while more than 40 per cent of teenage girls said they had already contemplated cosmetic surgery. See Decca Aitkenhead, 'Most British women Now Expect To Have Cosmetic Surgery in their Lifetime', *The Guardian* (14 September 2005). Also see 'Most Women "Want Plastic Surgery"', BBC *News Health* (8 August 2001).

2 Louis Uchitelle and N. R. Kleinfield, 'The Price of Jobs Lost', in *The Transformation of Work in the New Economy*, ed. R. Perrucci and C. C. Perrucci (Los Angeles, 2007), p. 84.

3 Dianna Solis, 'Plastic Surgery Wooing Patients Hoping To Move Up Career Ladder', *Wall Street Journal* (6 August 1985), p. 1.

4 Eryn Brown, 'Sometimes, Nips and Tucks Can Be Career Moves', *New York Times* (12 February 2006), pp. 3–6.

5 Diane E. Lewis, 'A New Wrinkle in the Rat Race', *Boston Globe* (7 June 2006), D1.

6 Paul Simao, 'Knife Guys Finish First', *Canadian Business*, LXIX/4 (April 1996), p. 121.

7 'Plastic Surgery Could Be the Key To Rejuvenating a Sagging Career', *Personnel Today* (25 April 2006), p. 9.

8 Suellen Hinde, '$20,000 Face Buys a New Job', *Sunday Mail* (10 June 2007), p. 24.

9 See J. Amman, T. Carpenter and G. Neff, eds, *Surviving the New Economy* (Boulder, CO, 2007). See also Perrucci and Perrucci, eds, *The Transformation of Work in the New Economy* (Oxford, 2007).

10 Richard Sennett, *The Culture of the New Capitalism* (New Haven, CT, 2006), p. 10.

Chapter 1: Drastic Plastic

1 Alex Kuczynski, *Beauty Junkies: Inside our $15 Billion Obsession with Cosmetic Surgery* (New York, 2006).

2 'Plastic Surgery Could Be the Key To Rejuvenating a Sagging Career',

Personnel Today (25 April 2006), p. 9.
3 David Bushnell, 'Personal Image as Business Strategy: Many Try To Gain an Edge by Fine-Tuning their Looks', *Boston Globe* (21 March 2004), G1.
4 Ferry Biedermann, 'Loans for Plastic Surgery Answer Lebanon's Yearning for Fresh Start', *Financial Times* (8 May 2007).
5 'Too Much: An Online Weekly on Excess and Inequality, October 8, 2007': www.cipa-apex.org/toomuch/Weeklies2007/Oct82007.html
6 Kuczynski, *Beauty Junkies*, p. 8;
7 Ariel Levy, *Female Chauvinist Pigs* (2006).
8 *Cosmetic Surgery Market Report 2007*, Key Note Publications, 2007, key1430689: www.marketresearch.com/product/print/default .asp?g=1&productid=1430689
9 Ibid.
10 Lisa Takeuchi Cullen, 'Changing Faces', *Time* (April 2006).
11 'China Likely To Become Asia's Plastic Surgery Centre', *Chinanews*: www.womenofchina.cn/focus/economy/3871.jsp
12 Fraser Newham, 'China Goes Under the Knife', *Asia Today* (8 June 2005): www.atimes.com/atimes/China/GF08Ad03.html
13 Barry Petersen, 'China Puts on a New Face', cbs *Evening News* (3 May 2005).
14 The exception here is the important socio-historical work of Sander Gilman, who has traced the interconnections among medicine, modernity, race and the surgically enhanced body. See Sander L. Gilman, *Making The Body Beautiful: A Cultural History of Aesthetic Surgery* (Princeton, NJ, 1999).
15 Naomi Wolf, *The Beauty Myth*.
16 Kathy Davis, *Reshaping the Female Body: The Dilemma of Cosmetic Surgery* (New York, 1995), p. 67.
17 Ibid., p. 5.
18 Virginia L. Blum, *Flesh Wounds: The Culture of Cosmetic Surgery* (Berkeley, CA, 2003), p. 56.
19 Ibid., p. 259.
20 Victoria Pitts-Taylor, *Surgery Junkies: Wellness and Pathology in Cosmetic Culture* (New Brunswick, NJ, 2007), p. 25.
21 Ibid., p. 165.
22 Anne Balsamo, *Technologies of the Gendered Body* (Durham, NC, 1996), p. 78.
23 Ibid., p. 58.
24 Suzanne Fraser, *Cosmetic Surgery, Gender and Culture* (London, 2003), p. 27.
25 Jill Scharff and Jaedene Levy, *The Facelift Diaries*, p. 12.
26 Kuczynski, *Beauty Junkies*, p. 7.
27 Ibid., p. 276.
28 Michael Zichy, 'Images of Man in the Discourse on Biotechnological Enhancement', paper presented at the conference *Engineering European Bodies: When Biomedical Technologies Challenge European Governance, Bioethics and Identities. University of Vienna, 14–16 June 2007*.
29 Natasha Singer, 'Q: Who Is the Real Face of Plastic Surgery?', *New York Times* (16 August 2007), Fashion and Style: 1.

30 On this point, see Anthony Giddens, *Modernity and Self-Identity* (Cambridge, 1991).

Chapter 2: Celebrity Obsession

1   Suellen Hinde, 'My Makeover Hell', *Adelaide Advertiser* (June 2007).
2   On the psychological and cultural intersections regarding the reduction of individuals to part-objects in porn, see Robert J. Stoller, *Porn* (New Haven, CT, 1993).
3   Leo Braudy, *The Frenzy of Renown* (New York, 1997).
4   Pamela Anderson quoted at www.bodylanguage.net/web/celebrity.html
5   Cher quoted at www.bodylanguage.net/web/celebrity.html
6   www.mtv.com/onair/i_want_a_famous_face/meet_the_patients_/index.jhtml?patients=Sha
7   Abigail Brooks, 'Under the Knife and Proud of It: An Analysis of the Normalization of Cosmetic Surgery', *Critical Sociology*, xxx/2 (2004), pp. 207–39.
8   Ibid., p. 225.
9   'Most Women "Want Plastic Surgery"', *BBC News Health* (8 August 2001): news.bbc.co.uk/2/hi/health/1480597.stm
10 Competition. http://news.bbc.co.uk/2/hi/entertainment/6390647.stm
11 Tamara McLean, 'Jolie Is Plastic Surgery "Gold Standard"' (12 April 2007): www.news.com.au/story/0,23599,21550173-36398,00.html
12 Richard Dyer, *Stars* (London, 1998), p. 39.
13 See Michel Foucault, *The Care of the Self* (London, 1986). See also Anthony Elliott, *Concepts of the Self*, 2nd edn (Cambridge, 2007), chapter 3.
14 Donald Horton and Richard Wohl, 'Mass Communications and Para-Social Interaction', *Psychiatry*, xix (1956), pp. 215–29; reprinted in *Communication Studies: An Introductory Reader*, ed. J. Corner and J. Hawthorne (London, 1993).
15 John B. Thompson, *The Media and Modernity* (Cambridge, 1995), p. 209.
16 See Anthony Elliott, *The Mourning of John Lennon* (Berkeley, CA, 1999).
17 Virginia L. Blum, *Flesh Wounds: The Culture of Cosmetic Surgery* (Berkeley, CA, 2003).
18 Sushi Das, 'Dear Doctor, Can You Make Me Look Like This Please?', *The Age* (10 March 2007), p. 3.
19 Ibid.
20 Margaret Gibson, 'Bodies without History: Cosmetic Surgery and the Undoing of Time', *Australian Feminist Studies*, xxi/49 (March 2006), p. 53.
21 Natasha Singer, 'And Thanks to My Agent, My Skin Doctor . . .', *New York Times* (18 February 2007), Fashion and Style, 1. The following quotation from Gary Lask is referenced from this article.
22 Gibson, 'Bodies without History', p. 52.
23 http://english.pravda.ru/society/showbiz/10-03-2006/77106-Madonna-0

24 John Gray, 'Ulrika Is a Sign That We've Got It All', *New Statesman* (28 October 2002), pp. 28–30.

Chapter 3: Want-Now Consumerism

1 Zygmunt Bauman, *Liquid Life* (Cambridge, 2005), p. 80.
2 Ibid., p. 77.
3 Ibid., p. 73.
4 Ibid., pp. 73–4.
5 Emine Saner, 'The Couple Who Spend 20K a Year on their Looks', *Evening Standard* (10 August 2005), pp. 21–2.
6 For a useful summary of recent social theories of consumerism, see Mark Patterson, *Consumption and Everyday Life* (London and New York, 2005).
7 Chris Schilling, *The Body and Society* (London, 2003).
8 The statistics provided here on surgical tourism are substantially informed by John Connell, 'Medical Tourism: Sea, Sun, Sand and . . . Surgery', *Journal of Tourism Management*, xxvii (2006), pp. 1093–100.
9 Ibid., p. 1095.
10 Ibid., p. 1094.
11 C. Levett, 'A Slice of the Action', *Sydney Morning Herald* (29 October 2005), p. 27.
12 Saskia Sassen, *Global Networks, Linked Cities* (London, 2002), p. 2.
13 John Urry, *Mobilities* (Cambridge, 2007), p. 152.
14 World Tourism Organization, *Yearbook of Tourist Statistics 2002* (Madrid, 2002).
15 John Urry, *Global Complexity* (Cambridge, 2003), pp. 1–2.
16 Mimi Sheller and John Urry, eds, *Tourism Mobilities* (London, 2004), p. 4.
17 M. Auge, *Non-Places* (London, 1995), pp. 75–9.
18 Doreen Massey, *Spatial Divisions of Labour* (London, 1984), p. 14.
19 M. Andrews, 'Vacation Makeovers', *us News and World Report* (19 January 2004).

Chapter 4: Making the Cut

1 Elizabeth Haiken, *Venus Envy: A History of Cosmetic Surgery* (Baltimore and London, 1997), p. 106.
2 Ibid., p. 107.
3 Eryn Brown, 'Sometimes Nips and Tucks Can Be Career Moves', *New York Times* (12 February 2006).
4 Ibid., Section 3, Part 6.
5 See Anthony Giddens, *Runaway World: How Globalization Is Reshaping our Lives* (London, 2003).
6 David Held, 'Democracy, the Nation-State and the Global System', *Economy and Society*, xx/2 (1991), p. 145. The more detailed version of this 'transformationalist' view of globalization is set out in D. Held et al., *Global Transformations* (Cambridge, 1999).

7 George Soros, *The Crisis of Global Capitalism: Open Society Endangered* (London, 1998).

8 Richard Sennett, *The Corrosion of Character* (New York, 1998), p. 23.

9 Richard Sennett, *The Culture of the New Capitalism* (New Haven, CT, 2005), p. 132.

10 Ibid., p. 141.

11 Gene Grossman and Esteban Rossi-Hansberg, 'The Rise of Offshoring: It's Not Wine for Cloth Anymore', in *The New Economic Geography: Effects and Policy Implications* (Kansas City, MO, 2006) pp. 59–102.

12 Zygmunt Bauman, *Wasted Lives: Modernity and its Outcasts* (Cambridge, 2004), p. 128.

13 Ibid.

14 Ibid.

15 Ibid., p. 106.

16 See Anthony Elliott, ed., *The Contemporary Bauman* (London and New York, 2007).

17 'Men Try To Put a New Face on Careers', *Wall Street Journal* (28 August 1991), p. B1. The subsequent quotes in this paragraph are taken from this article.

18 'Plastic That Is Not Necessarily So Fantastic', *Financial Times* (13 March 1999), Body and Mind Section, p. 2.

19 'Spanish Group Seeks Facelift with Flotation', *Financial Times* (23 May 2005), p. 23. Subsequent quotations in this paragraph are from this article.

20 'One in Four Executive Women Would Consider Cosmetic Surgery', *M2 Presswire* [Coventry] (30 May 2005), p. 1.

21 Sigmund Freud, 'Inhibitions, Symptoms and Anxiety' 1925, in *The Standard Edition of the Complete Psychological Works of Sigmund Freud*, ed. James Strachey, 24 vols (London 1953–74), vol. XX, p. 170. The infant, it seems, relies on the mother in a profoundly imaginary way: through the medium of fantasy, constructions of self and other, sameness and difference become possible. The forging of some preliminary sense of identity, Freud argues, arises through an imagined incorporation of the mother into the self. In effect, Freud argues that what is on the outside (the body of the mother) can be taken inside (psychic space), internalized and devoured. Our primary experiences with the mother become part of the emotional structure of subjectivity.

22 Sigmund Freud, 'Mourning and Melancholia' [1915], in *The Standard Edition of the Complete Psychological Works of Sigmund Freud*, ed. James Strachey, 24 vols (London, 1953–74), vol. XIV, p. 251. For a discussion of the centrality of mourning to psychoanalysis, see Madelon Sprengnether, 'Mourning Freud', in *Psychoanalysis in Contexts: Paths between Theory and Modern Culture*, ed. Anthony Elliott and Stephen Frosh (London, 1995), pp. 142–65. See also Peter Homans, *The Ability to Mourn* (Chicago, IL, 1989).

23 The shift from the process of mourning to that of melancholia involves acute narcissistic depression. Projective identification and incorporation, as Melanie Klein has shown, give the fantasized dimensions of this idealization and valourization of self / other

merging. Klein describes the object relation as structured by a paranoid, schizoid position. This is a schizoid splitting that underpins the integration of the subject (the division between the 'good' and 'bad' mother), but it is also linked to a logics of fragmentation in which the subject imagines itself disintegrating into pieces. See Melanie Klein, 'A Contribution to the Psychogenesis of Manic-Depressive States' and 'Mourning and Its Relation to Manic-Depressive States', in Melanie Klein, *Love, Guilt and Reparation and Other Works, 1921–1945* (London, 1988), pp. 262–89 and 334–69.

24 In the psychoanalytic frame of reference, loss lies at the foundation of personal and social life. The Freudian Oedipus complex, as the French psychoanalyst Jacques Lacan has emphasized, accounts for the dissolution of the child's narcissistic omnipotence and his or her insertion into the law-governed world of language and symbols. After Oedipus, the individual lives out a symbolic relationship to loss in and through an object world of introjects and identifications. But the negotiation of loss depends on the ability to mourn, an ability that is profoundly disrupted and disturbed with the advent of melancholia. See Jacques Lacan, 'The Agency of the Letter in the Unconscious of Reason since Freud', *Ecrits* (London, 1977), chapter 5. For a critical appraisal of Lacan's return to Freud, see Anthony Elliott, *Social Theory and Psychoanalysis in Transition* (Oxford, 1992), chapter 4.

25 Julia Kristeva, *Black Sun: Depression and Melancholia* (New York, 1989), p. 6.

26 Don DeLillo, *Underworld* (London, 1998), p. 786.

27 Shelley Gare, 'Do You Think I'm Sixty?', *Australian Weekend Magazine* (7–8 April 2007), p. 16.

28 Margaret Gibson, 'Bodies without History: Cosmetic Surgery and the Undoing of Time', *Australian Feminist Studies*, xxi/49 (March 2006), p. 55.

29 Julia Kristeva, *Power of Horror* (New York, 1982).

30 Maurice Blanchot, *L'Entretien infini* (Paris, 1969), pp. 269–70.

31 See Anthony Giddens, *Modernity and Self-Identity* (Cambridge, 1991).

32 Alan Kellehear, *A Social History of Dying* (Cambridge, 2006), p. 253.

33 Terry Eagleton, *After Theory* (London, 2003), p. 213.

34 Jeff Edwards and Emily Miller, 'Dad Held as Girl, 2, Has Skull Smashed', *Daily Mirror* (4 June 2007), p. 1. I have also drawn details from Duncan Gardham, 'Girl, 2, Beaten after Disturbing Morning Lie-in', *Daily Telegraph* (6 June 2007), p. 1.

Acknowledgements

This book began around the time of the completion of *The New Individualism*, an investigation of the emotional costs of globalization. I learned a great deal about the short-termism of the global economy from Charles Lemert – which I have been able to apply in this study. His commitment to the practical and public import of sociology has inspired my research, and I dedicate this book to him.

Various public forums and institutions afforded me the opportunity to try out ideas (sometimes half-raw) for this book. Of crucial importance were the dialogues and debates with audiences at the Tate Modern, London, 2005; the Watershed Media Centre, Bristol, 2006; the ESRC Identities and Social Action Programme, Birmingham, 2006; the South Australian Art Gallery, Adelaide, 2006; the Australian Sociological Association Conference, Perth, 2006; and the Brisbane Writers Festival, 2007. I have also spoken on cosmetic surgical culture at various universities, including Vienna, the London School of Economics, University College Dublin, Exeter, Glasgow Caledonian University and Nottingham.

I should like to thank the numerous cosmetic surgeons and patients who gave so freely of their time to this project. I have sought to disguise their identities in order to protect confidentially, and (as with *The New Individualism*) deploy the method of fictionalized case-narratives as detailed in the Introduction. I am grateful to all of those who agreed to be interviewed for this project, and especially for the various kinds of insight and feedback that allowed me to pull together the social theory and cultural criticism about cosmetic surgical culture that I'd done over recent years.

The Department of Sociology at Flinders University has been a superb intellectual environment in which to complete my research, and I wish to thank in particular my students in the Flinders Social Theory Group. In this connection, Daniel Chaffee and Eric Hsu deserve particular mention for their intellectual support and assistance with various practical matters. Expert research assistance at Flinders was also provided by Carolyn Corkindale. In addition, the Department of Sociology at the Open University afforded me the time, through a Visiting Research Professorship, to complete work on developments in cosmetic surgical culture in the UK and Europe.

I'd like to thank Vivian Constantinopoulos of Reaktion Books. Special thanks to colleagues and friends with whom I've discussed aspects of this book, especially Anthony Moran, Gerhard Boomgaarden, Paul du Gay, Fiore Inglese, Alison Assiter, Paul Hoggett, Kriss McKie, Deborah Maxwell and Jem Thomas. I'd especially like to thank Nicola Geraghty – along with Caoimhe, Oscar and Niamh – for the many ways in which they supported the work, urging me to say what I had to say to the widest possible audience, and above all to get the book finished. Against the backdrop of moving from Bristol to Canterbury to Adelaide, this might have been considered something of a tall order – but with their emotional support and love, it seemed easy.

Photo Acknowledgements

The author and publishers wish to express their thanks to the following source of illustrative material and permission to reproduce it:

Photos courtesy Rex Features: pp. 14 (Bernadete Lou/Rex Features, 374546M), 48 (Stewart Cook/Rex Features, 617511AI), 78 (Fotex/Rex Features, 701598A), 108 (Image Source/Rex Features, 509569A).